传播中医药文化
架设东西方桥梁

范永升

2021. 5. 18

首届全国名中医
"973"首席科学家
浙江中医药大学原校长

浙江省社科联社科普及课题成果（18ZZ02）

# 探访中医药文化：汉英对照

ZHEJIANG UNIVERSITY PRESS
浙江大学出版社

**图书在版编目（CIP）数据**

探访中医药文化：汉英对照 / 梁世伟主编. — 杭
州：浙江大学出版社，2021.6
ISBN 978-7-308-21410-0

Ⅰ. ①探… Ⅱ. ①梁… Ⅲ. ①中国医药学－文化－
汉、英 Ⅳ. ①R2-05

中国版本图书馆CIP数据核字(2021)第099834号

**探访中医药文化：汉英对照**

梁世伟　主编

| | |
|---|---|
| **责任编辑** | 殷晓彤　徐有智 |
| **责任校对** | 金佩雯 |
| **封面设计** | 余里豪 |
| **出版发行** | 浙江大学出版社 |
| | （杭州市天目山路148号　　邮政编码　310007） |
| | （网址：http://www.zjupress.com） |
| **排　　版** | 杭州林智广告有限公司 |
| **印　　刷** | 杭州良诸印刷有限公司 |
| **开　　本** | 880mm×1230mm　1/32 |
| **印　　张** | 8 |
| **字　　数** | 200千 |
| **版 印 次** | 2021年6月第1版　2021年6月第1次印刷 |
| **书　　号** | ISBN 978-7-308-21410-0 |
| **定　　价** | 49.00元 |

# 《探访中医药文化：汉英对照》

# 编 委 会

主 审：项隆元

主 编：梁世伟

副主编：梁泽华　张国利　林　洁

编 委：徐宁骏　叶　晓　袁慧玲

　　　　李　彤　扈李娟　唐　路

# 前　言

　　中华文化是中华各族人民在社会历史发展过程中所创造的物质文化和精神文化的总和，而中医药文化是中华优秀传统文化的重要组成部分，体现了中华优秀传统文化的核心价值观和思维方式。中医药文化指中医学理论体系形成的社会文化背景以及蕴含的人文价值和文化特征，包括物质层面、行为层面、精神层面的文化内涵。中医药在发展过程中，为后人留下了浩如烟海的中医古籍文献、难以计数的诊疗器物、各种特色的医疗场所等，构筑了中医绚丽多彩的物质文化，表明了我国传统医学文化的博大精深，为我们展现了一幅幅古代中医药的生动图景。行为文化层面可以让我们窥探中医药文化的核心价值观在中医药从业者行为上的具体体现。中医的精神层面包括中医的价值观念和思维方式。中医价值观主要体现在天人观、生命观、疾病观、治疗观、养生观和道德观；而中医的思维方式具有象数思维、整体思维、体悟思维的特点。两者共同从根本上规定了中医的基本理论和诊疗方式。

　　为了在广大海内外喜爱中医药文化的非中医药专业人群普及中医药文化，根据中医药文化的三个层面的特点，发现、体验、感悟中医药文化是个实用、易实践的办法，如：参观中医药博物馆、中医药老字号；学太极拳、接受中药或针灸治疗、学做药膳、品鉴传统食物中的中医药文化、体验养生保健；探寻和感悟中医药古代文化、理解成语典故、感悟历代医家的德高医湛等。

因此，在浙江省社科联社科普及课题项目（18ZZ02）的支持下，我们整理编辑了一些简短、朗朗上口的中文小文章，并将其翻译成英文。本书集科普性、语言学习于一体，以接受新事物的基本生理规律，从视觉上发现、从身体上体验、从思维中感悟，通过看到、参与、领悟生活中的中医药文化，进而引发读者对中医药文化的好奇心。

本书的目的是普及中医药文化、唤起读者兴趣，所以本书不是对某一中医药文化的详细介绍与研究而是科普介绍，由博反约，深入浅出，直白有趣，说好中医故事。本书读者可以是在校修习中医学课程的学生、广大的中医药文化爱好者及来华学习的留学生等。

本书从以下几个部分展开科普性中英文介绍：上篇发现篇，分为中医药老字号、中医药博物馆、药用植物园三个章节，对陈李济中药博物馆、潘高寿、九芝堂、鹤年堂、同仁堂、胡庆余堂、长春堂、广誉远、北京中医药大学中医药博物馆、上海中医药博物馆、藏医药文化博物馆、国家图书馆之甲骨文、北京故宫博物院之《清明上河图》以及药用植物园等作科普性介绍。中篇体验篇分为养生观概论、饮食养生、起居养生、运动养生、治疗养生五个章节，对养生的种类及各种具体的养生体验作科普性介绍。下篇感悟篇分为考古文物、神医名医、成语故事、象征符号、历史痕迹五个章节，发掘蕴藏在各种事物与现象中的中医药文化内涵。通过介绍中医药文化的各种现象，尝试为继承传统文化、挖掘中医药历史价值、开拓新时代的中医药文化、增进国际交流增添一份力量。

本书的编写是伴随着《中医文化（双语）》的课堂教学知识的凝练而产生的。为了给学生提供丰富的中医药文化知识，编者查阅了大量的文献资料、网络信息资源、公众平台信息资源。在写作和整理过程中，自己也得到了学习和提升，深感中医药古代文化的魅力和博大精深。编者带着强大的责任感和浓厚的中医药文化情结，花了近两年时间完成此书的编写和翻译。在此过程中，得到了家人、同事、教育界大咖以及浙江大学出版社的帮助和支持，借此表示由衷的感谢。正是大家的热心帮助和支持，才使这本书得以顺利付梓。

由于作者水平有限，不当与错误之处恐难免，恳请读者与同道提出宝贵意见，以便再版时修订。

梁世伟

2021年6月于杭州西子湖畔

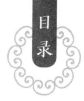

中篇

# 体验篇

## PART II

## EXPERIENCE

# 感悟篇
## PART III
## GNOSIS

上篇

发现篇

PART I
DISCOVERY

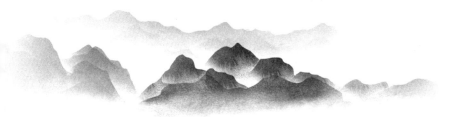

# 老字号与老字号博物馆
## Time-honored Brands and Museums

## 第一节　陈李济中药博物馆
### Chenliji Museum of Chinese Medicine

　　陈李济中药博物馆是由广州老字号陈李济开办的博物馆，也是岭南地区首家中药行业博物馆。作为中医药400年的鲜活记录，陈李济中药博物馆以场景复原形式，向参观者展现中药传统工艺。陈李济成功地将蜂蜡与木蜡混合，制成了既不软也不硬的蜡壳，用来包裹药丸，带来了医药制剂领域的巨大革新。在制作蜡丸初期，陈李济还创立了独特的陈皮储藏方法。陈皮体轻、气味清香，久煮不烂，对祛风化痰有绝佳疗效，放置百年也不会有虫霉变，有"百年陈皮胜黄金"的说法。据资料记载，如今陈列在展厅中的镇馆之宝——陈皮，已有百余年历史，伴随着陈李济从清朝一路走来，是无价之宝。陈皮储存需年年翻晒，百年陈皮承载了多少代陈李济人对于中药的执着。陈李济是由陈姓商人和李姓医生共同出资创立的，店名含有二人的姓以表示永远合作，同心济世。几百年前，陈李济订下规矩，凡是路过门市者，一旦晕倒或受伤，必施药相救。在这里，百年的文物、医药古籍原本、名贵的药材以及宝物不计其数，当然还有更多的故事讲不尽、道不完。

Chenliji Museum of Chinese Medicine, the first museum of Chinese medicine industry in Lingnan area, was established by a time-honored brand Chenliji in Guangzhou. As a living record of 400 years of traditional Chinese medicine (TCM), Chenliji Museum of Chinese Medicine focuses on scene restoration to show visitors the traditional techniques of Chinese medicine. Chenliji revolutionized the field of pharmaceutical preparations by successfully mixing beeswax with wood wax to make a wax shell that was neither soft nor hard to wrap around pills. It also developed a unique way to store tangerine peel when it first made the pellets. The tangerine peel is light with a fragrant smell. If decocted for long, it is not squishy. It has excellent efficacy of dispelling wind and phlegm. After preserved for a hundred years, it would not go mouldy, proving a saying that "hundred years of tangerine peel is more valuable than gold". Now displayed in the exhibition hall, the most treasured piece, the tangerine peel, according to records, has been stored for more than a hundred years, which is priceless. It has accompanied Chenliji all the way from the Qing Dynasty. The storage of the tangerine peel requires annual drying. The century-old tangerine peel bears the dedication of many generations of Chenliji people to TCM. Chenliji was jointly founded by a merchant surnamed Chen and a doctor surnamed Li. They took their own family name together, indicating that they would work together forever to help those in need. For hundreds of years, Chenliji has made a rule that if anyone passing by the pharmacy fainted or was injured, Chenliji would give medicine to help him. Here, the century-old cultural relics, ancient medical books, rare medicinal materials as well as treasures are countless and many stories about them can be told endlessly.

## 第二节　潘高寿
**Pan'gaoshou**

　　1890年，潘百世、潘应世兄弟在广州开设药铺"长春洞"。之后，潘百世的四子潘郁生根据岭南独特的气候特征，将具有润肺镇咳作用的川贝母和有祛痰作用的桔梗与枇杷叶一起熬炼，于1928年制成了止咳化痰的新药，名为"潘高寿川贝枇杷露"。潘高寿一直采用传统方式生产：煮药用的是铁锅木柴、土炉明火，跟民间"煲凉茶"一样。浓缩药液和煮糖也是用明火煎熬，木棍搅拌。由于怕配方泄露，调配药液往往是药铺老板亲自动手，或者叫自己的亲戚做配药。作为"中华老字号"的潘高寿，首创独特的川贝枇杷露制作工艺，突出体现了立足传统、大胆革新的岭南医药文化特征。因为潘高寿对高品质原材料的把关以及制作工艺流程的严格控制，所以潘高寿在止咳药行业里成为一枝独秀，是中国本土止咳药最突出的代表之一。同时，潘高寿又集中体现了岭南商业文化的特征，是目前已知的岭南地区最早的维护知识产权的百年老店之一。

　　In 1890, brothers Pan Baishi and Pan Yingshi opened a pharmacy named "Changchun Cave" in Guangzhou. Later, Pan Yusheng, the fourth son of Pan Baishi, refined bulbus fritillaria cirrhosa, which had the effect of nourishing the lung and suppressing cough, and the root of platycodon grandiflorus, which had the effect of removing phlegm together with loquat leaves. In 1928, a new medicine for relieving cough and reducing phlegm was made and named as "Pan'gaoshou Syrup of Tendril-leaved Fritillary Bulb and Loquat". The pharmacy has been using the traditional way of production: iron pot and wood are used for decocting medicine with clay stoves and naked fire, imitating the folk people to cook herbal tea. Concentrated medicine and boiled sugar are also cooked over an open fire and stirred with wooden sticks. For fear of betraying the formula, the dispensing of liquid medicine is often either done by the boss himself or their relatives. As a "China Time-honored Brand", Pan'gaoshou pioneered the unique production technology of Syrup of Tendril-leaved Fritillary Bulb and Loquat, which highlighted the characteristics of Lingnan medical culture based on tradition and bold innovation. The control of high-quality raw materials and strict production process have made Pan'gaoshou a standout in the cough medicine industry, making it the most prominent representative of the local cough medicine in China. At the same time, Pan'gaoshou embodies the characteristics of Lingnan commercial culture. It is one of the earliest known century-old pharmacies in Lingnan that maintains intellectual property rights.

## 第三节　九芝堂
### Jiuzhi Hall

　　清顺治七年（1650年），劳澄在湖南长沙创建了九芝堂。劳澄在创建初期就仿效神农氏亲自试药，立下了"吾药必吾先尝之"的规矩，为九芝堂中药文化奠定了最初范型。在发展壮大过程中，九芝堂发扬了湖湘文化中的"敢为人先"和"经世致用"的精神，传承"悬壶济世，利泽生民"的湖湘中医药文化精髓，将传统的中药制药技术与湖南当地水土环境结合，形成了九芝堂特有的"药者当付全力，医者当问良心"的人文精神。经世代相传，已成为九芝堂人的行为准则，并成为传统中医药文化的一部分。九芝堂将传统中药炮制技术和传统制剂技术加以完善和提高，它代表了湖湘传统中药制药技术和方法的较高标准和水平。九芝堂的"恤苦济贫，优益同业""扶危救人""重质量，讲诚信""九分情，一分利"的经营理念对医药行业的发展具有重要的促进作用。弘扬九芝堂传统中药文化，对于弘扬祖国优秀的中医药文化具有重要推动作用。

　　In 1650, the 7th year of Shunzhi in the Qing Dynasty, Lao Cheng established Jiuzhi Hall in Changsha, Hunan Province. At the early stage of its establishment, Lao Cheng imitated Shennong to taste medicine in person and established the rule that "I must taste the medicine first", which laid the initial model for the TCM culture of Jiuzhi Hall. Later, Jiuzhi Hall carried forward the spirit of "daring to be the first" and "serving the public" in Xiang culture. It inherits the essence of Hunan TCM culture, which is "helping the world and benefiting the people", combines the TCM pharmaceutical technology with the local water and soil environment in Hunan and forms the unique humanistic spirit of Jiuzhi Hall, which is "the drug-makers should pay their best and the doctors should have conscience". Through generations, the ancestral motto has become a code of conduct for Jiuzhi Hall people and a part of TCM culture. Jiuzhi Hall has perfected and improved the herbal processing technology and traditional preparation technology, which represents the high standard and level of pharmaceutical technology and methods of Chinese medicine in Hunan. Jiuzhi Hall's business philosophy of "helping the poor, benefiting the industry", "helping and saving people in emergency", "focusing on quality and integrity", "ninety percent of benevolence and ten percent of profit" has played an important role in promoting the development of the pharmaceutical industry. To carry forward the TCM culture of Jiuzhi Hall plays an important role in promoting the excellent Chinese medicine culture of the motherland.

# 第四节　鹤年堂
## Henian Hall

北京鹤年堂于1405年成立，至今已有600多年的历史。明清时期，鹤年堂为皇宫配制药膳、养生酒、茶等养生用品。鹤年堂制药坚持"精选上品"和"精心炮制"，得到人们的一致好评。清朝皇族和喜欢吃滋补药品的南方人多在鹤年堂买药。鹤年堂的药材饮片采用分别包装的办法，每一品种的包装内都放有"图说内票"，票上印有药名、产地、气味、主治何病和药的图形。顾客把药抓回去，可对照说明查对。鹤年堂的名声不仅源于它高品质的药材，更因它与多位名人的趣闻轶事有关。戚继光作为我国历史上的民族英雄，有一次他率军征战归来，最先前往的地方竟然就是鹤年堂。因为在征战中将士们受刀枪所伤，再加上南方沿海地区气候湿热，时时受到瘟疫的威胁。鹤年堂为戚家军送去了精心研制的"白鹤保命丹"等急救药、刀伤药和避瘟药，挽救了许多将士的生命。数百年来，鹤年堂坚持"生身以养寿为先，养身以却病为急"的理念，形成了以"调元气，养太和"为文化内涵的鹤年堂中医药养生文化。

Founded in 1405, Henian Hall in Beijing has a history of more than 600 years. In the Ming and Qing Dynasties, Henian Hall prepared medicinal meals, medicated liquor, tea and other health care products for the imperial palace. Henian Hall gets people's unanimous praise by adhering to the "selection for high-quality raw materials" and "careful processing" as their pharmaceutical essence. The royal families of the Qing Dynasty and southerners who liked to take tonic medicine mostly bought medicine in Henian Hall. The medicinal materials here were packed separately with an "illustration" for each, on which the name of the medicine, the place of origin, the property and flavor, indications and the picture of the medicine were printed. When the customers took the medicine home, they could check it according to the instructions. Henian Hall is famous not only for the high quality of its medicine, but also for its anecdotes about some famous people. Qi Jiguang is a national hero in the history of our country. Once he returned from a war with his army, the first place he visited was Henian Hall. It turned out that during the war, the soldiers were inevitably wounded by swords and guns, and threatened by pestilence from time to time due to the hot and humid climate in the southern coastal areas. Henian Hall sent carefully produced "Pellets for Preserving life", wound medicine, anti-plague medicine and other first-aid medicines for Qi's army, saving many soldiers' lives. For hundreds of years, Henian Hall has always been adhering to the concept of "taking care of life first and taking care of health as the urgent", forming the TCM health culture with the cultural connotation of "regulating vitality and purchasing supreme harmony".

# 第五节　同仁堂
## Tongren Hall

　　北京同仁堂创建于1669年，自1723年开始供奉御药，历经八代皇帝188年。在300多年的风雨历程中，历代同仁堂人始终恪守"炮制虽繁必不敢省人工，品味虽贵必不敢减物力"的古训，树立了"修合无人见，存心有天知"的自律精神，形成了制药过程中兢兢业业、精益求精的风格，其产品以"配方独特、选料上乘、工艺精湛、疗效显著"而享誉海内外。同仁堂创建人是乐家第四代乐尊育先生，乐家祖上都是走街串巷的行医卖药人。清康熙八年（1669年），乐尊育创办了同仁堂药室。同仁堂的中成药以用药地道、加工精致而闻名全国。据说在同仁堂的库房里有人发现了150多年前留存的一批成药，大家都以为这批药应该早已发霉变质了，可是剥开来一看，粒粒香气浓郁，黑里透光，经过鉴定，药力不减，说明该店出品的药物，质量非常过硬。百年药铺之所以长兴不衰，这与其坚持艰苦创业的精神，后继人才的恪守祖业、勇于进取、经营得法、善于管理，并懂得任人唯贤，是分不开的。

　　Tongren Hall in Beijing was founded in 1669 and has been offering royal medicine since 1723. It has served eight generations of emperors for 188 years. For more than 300 years of ups and downs, all the previous founders and owners have always been adhering to the old adage that "although the processing is cumbersome, labor should not be saved and although high-grade medicine is expensive, we must not ignore the quality of raw materials". They have set up the self-discipline consciousness of "no going against your conscience and being honest to customers without supervision" and created the meticulous spirit of care and excellence in the pharmaceutical process. Its products are famous at home and abroad for their unique formula, superior material selection, exquisite workmanship and remarkable curative effect. Tongren Hall's founder was the fourth generation Le Zunyu whose previous generations were all itinerant practitioners and drug sellers. In the eighth year of the reign of Emperor Kangxi of the Qing Dynasty (1669 A.D.), Le Zunyu established the Tongren Hall pharmacy. Its proprietary Chinese medicines are famous for their authentic uses and exquisite processing. A true story tells us that a batch of prepared medicines preserved over 150 years ago were found in the storeroom of Tongren Hall. Everyone thought that these medicines had long been moldy and deteriorated. However, when peeled off, they showed strong aroma, transparent light in the dark and the efficacy of the medicines remained unchanged after identification, indicating that the quality of the medicines produced by the store was excellent. The reason why the century-old pharmaceutical store has been flourishing is that it is inseparable from the spirit of hard work, the people who abide by the ancestral business with the courage to forge ahead, the skills and experience of operation and management and the knowledge of appointing people to their merits.

老字号与老字号博物馆 第一章

## 第六节　胡庆余堂
**Huqingyu Hall**

　　胡庆余堂，由清末胡雪岩于1874年创建，地处杭州历史文化街区清河坊，是国内保存最完好的晚清工商型古建筑群。整个药店的格局是传统的前店后厂，前面是营业大厅，后面是制药作坊。门楼上至今还保留着创始人胡雪岩所立"是乃仁术"四个大字，表达了胡雪岩创办药店济世救人的初衷。传统建筑的匾额一般是朝外挂的，但胡庆余堂有一块最出名的匾额则是朝里，面向坐堂经理的方向挂着的，上书"戒欺"二字和一篇胡雪岩手书的谆谆教诲，告诫药店的员工药业关系性命，万不可欺。营业大厅现在已成为胡庆余堂中药博物馆的陈列厅，展示着古代的制药工具等文物。胡庆余堂资本雄厚，采购各种名贵药材和道地药材可谓不遗余力。为了求得上品药材，胡庆余堂常常提前一年借钱给药农，使他们预先周转，药农们自然用上品相售。胡庆余堂数次易主，但药店的名号始终未变，被视为胡雪岩经营最为成功的企业。这成功的背后，仁爱和诚信的中国传统商业精神，精明的商业头脑和广告宣传策略，可谓缺一不可。

Huqingyu Hall, founded by Hu Xueyan in 1874 A.D. in the late Qing Dynasty, is located in Qinghefang, a historical and cultural block in Hangzhou. It is the best-preserved industrial and commercial ancient architectural complex in the late Qing Dynasty in China. The pattern of the whole pharmacy is the shop in front and the factory at the back, namely, the front is the business hall and the back is the pharmaceutical workshop. On the gate, there are four characters showing the implication of "making drugs is closely related with benevolence and skills" written by the founder Hu Xueyan, which expresses the original intention of Hu Xueyan to set up the pharmacy to benefit the people. Traditional building plaques are generally hung outward, but Huqingyu Hall has one of the most famous plaques hung inward, which reads "Quit cheating" and a manuscript of Hu Xueyan, telling the pharmacy staff that drugs are a matter of life and people should never be cheated. The business hall has now become the exhibition hall of Huqingyu Hall of Museum of Chinese Medicine, displaying ancient pharmaceutical tools and other cultural relics. With abundant capital, Huqingyu Hall has spared no effort in purchasing all kinds of rare and authentic medicinal materials. In order to obtain high-quality medicinal materials, Huqingyu Hall lent the farmers money often a year in advance, so that the farmers had capital turnover and naturally provided high-quality materials. Huqingyu Hall has changed its owners several times, but the name of the pharmacy hasn't been changed, which is regarded as the most successful business operated by Hu Xueyan. Behind this success, benevolence and integrity as the business morality, shrewd business mind and advertising strategy can be said to be indispensable.

## 第七节 长春堂
**Changchun Hall**

清乾隆年间，北京有位走街串巷的游方郎中，名叫孙振兰，在前门大街鲜鱼口胡同里置了间铺房，挂上了"长春堂"的字号，开始了前店后厂，固定经营的方式，结束了游方郎中的生活，这就是长春堂的创始老店。长春堂药店于1795年开张营业，距今已有200多年的历史。说到"长春堂"，老北京人马上会想起"避瘟散"。1888年，孙三明开始经营长春堂。为了与日本产的仁丹和清凉闻药宝丹相抗衡，他潜心钻研，经过十年努力最终试制成功了一种新的闻药——避瘟散。1933年左右，避瘟散终于取代了日货宝丹而独占市场。其中，1933年销售达250万盒，以华北、华东销售量最大，同时在泰国、印尼、缅甸等国都有销售。这一时期应该说是长春堂的鼎盛时期。消暑闻药避瘟散具有香、凉、祛瘟消暑的功效，取用少许抹入鼻腔，清凉之感直通心脑。1996年，长春堂拥有中西药批发零售、中医医馆、代客邮寄等业务，荣获国家授予的"中华老字号"称号。时至今日，盛夏时节到长春堂购买避瘟散的顾客仍旧络绎不绝。

During the reign of Emperor Qianlong of the Qing Dynasty, an itinerant doctor, named Sun Zhenlan, set up a pharmacy in Xianyukou Hutong, Qianmen Street and put up the name of

"Changchun Hall". The fixed business mode of "front shop and back factory" ended his itinerant life, which was the founding old shop of Changchun Hall. Changchun Hall pharmacy was open in 1795 with a history of more than 200 years. When it comes to "Changchun Hall", old Beijingers will think of "the powder for avoiding plague". In 1888, Sun Sanming began to run Changchun Hall. In order to compete with ren pillets and treasured pillets for cooling, two Japanese products, he devoted himself to research. After ten years of efforts he successfully produced a new olfactory medicine — the powder for avoiding plague. By 1933 or so, the powder finally had replaced the Japanese treasured pillets and monopolized the market. In 1933, 2.5 million boxes were sold with the largest sales volume in Northern and Eastern China. At the same time in Thailand, Indonesia, Myanmar and other countries markets came into being. This period was the peak of Changchun Hall. Such an olfactory drug as the powder for avoiding fever has the fragrant effect of cooling, dispelling fever and dissipating heat. Take a little and wipe it into the nasal cavity and the cool feeling goes straight to the chest and head. In 1996, Changchun Hall owned the business of wholesale and retail of Chinese and western medicine, Chinese medicine clinic and mail for customers. It was awarded "China Time-honored Brand" by the government. Today, the customers who go to Changchun Hall to buy the olfactory powder in summer are still coming in an endless stream.

老字号与老字号博物馆　第一章

## 第八节　广誉远
### Guangyuyuan

　　山西省广誉远中药有限公司是我国现存历史最悠久的中药企业，它的前身广盛号药店始创于明嘉靖二十年（1541年）。在清代，山西广誉远与广州陈李济（1600年建立）、北京同仁堂（1669年建立）、杭州胡庆余堂（1874年建立）并称为"清代四大药店"。2006年，广誉远成为首批被国家商务部认定的"中华老字号"企业。据太平天国史料记载，太平天国攻克南京后，天王洪秀全曾密令要将广盛药号店全部迁往南京。广盛号药店当时的地位由此可见一斑。广誉远拥有丰富的产品，有丸剂、胶囊剂、酒剂、片剂、颗粒剂、散剂、口服液、煎膏剂共八个剂型，继承着龟龄集、定坤丹、安宫牛黄丸、牛黄清心丸、六味地黄丸、乌鸡白凤丸等103种中药古方及炮制工艺，从方剂、配伍、选材、炮制等诸多方面，承载并展现着中医药文化的核心精神与巨大价值。历代广誉远人恪守诚实敬业的品德，将"修合虽无人见，存心自有天知"作为生产药品的信条，养成了良好的自律精神。这种精神在今天最直接的体现就是良心制药。

　　Shanxi Guangyuyuan Chinese Medicine Co., Ltd. is the oldest existing Chinese medicine enterprise in China. Its predecessor, Guangsheng Pharmacy, was founded in 1541 A.D. in the 20th year of Jiajing in the Ming Dynasty. In the Qing Dynasty, Shanxi Guangyuyuan, along with Chenliji in Guangzhou (established in 1600), Tongren Hall in Beijing (established in 1669) and Huqingyu Hall in Hangzhou (established in 1874), were known as the "Four Great Drugstores of the Qing Dynasty". In 2006, it became one of the first "time-honored" enterprises recognized by the Ministry of Commerce, PRC. According to the historical records of the Taiping Heavenly Kingdom, after the Taiping Heavenly Kingdom conquered Nanjing, the King Hong Xiuquan secretly ordered all Guangsheng pharmacies to be moved to Nanjing. It shows the significance of Guangsheng Pharmacy at that time. Guangyuyuan has a wealth of products such as pills, capsules, medicinal liquor, tablets, granules, powder and oral liquid. It inherits Guilingji, Dingkun Pellets, and Niuhuang Pills for Protecting Uterus, Niuhuang Pills for Clearing the Heart Fire, Liuwei Dihuang Pills, Wuji Baifeng Pills and other 103 kinds of prescriptions and processing techniques. It carries and shows the core spirit and great value of TCM culture from the aspects of prescription, compatibility, material selection and processing. In the past dynasties, people of Guangyuyuan scrupulously abided by honesty and dedication and took "no going against your conscience and being honest to customers without supervision" as the credo of drug production and developed a good self-discipline spirit. The most direct manifestation of this spirit today is pharmaceutical conscience.

# 博物馆
## Museums

## 第一节　北京中医药大学中医药博物馆
### Museum of Traditional Chinese Medicine, Beijing University of Chinese Medicine

北京中医药大学中医药博物馆展出医药文物、塑像、模型、绘画、拓片、照片、医药用具、古医书等1000余种。共收藏历代医史文物930余件、古代线装医籍200余种、中医书刊6000余册，其中有扁鹊行医图（汉代画像石）、历代名医塑像、沙盘模型、仿清光绪时期的针灸铜人、少数民族医药用具、明代医药书籍等。镇馆之宝是仿宋针灸铜人，是南京博物院按照清代光绪年间太医院的铜人复制的。太医院复制的铜人曾经随着国家的命运几经辗转，先后于1925年移交故宫博物院，于1933年春随同第三批文物南迁，移交南京博物院，于1958年回到中国历史博物馆。据说太医院复制的铜人是仿制北宋著名医家王惟一铸造的天圣铜人，但世事沧桑，王惟一亲手铸造的两具铜人，最终不知去向。在古代，针灸铜人像被用作教学和考试。具体做法是，先在铜人体表涂满黄蜡，然后向其体内灌满水。当学生刺中穴位时，水就会从穴位处流出。如果不中，针则刺不进去。这样，老师就可以准确地判断学生的学习情况了。

Museum of Traditional Chinese Medicine of Beijing University of Chinese Medicine exhibits more than 1,000 kinds of medical relics, statues, models, paintings, rubbings, photographs, medical appliances, ancient medical books and so on. The museum has a total collection of more than 930 pieces of historical medical relics, more than 200 kinds of ancient thread-bound medical books, and more than 6,000 books and periodicals of TCM, including Bian Que's medical practice pictures (engraved on stone in the Han Dynasty), famous doctors of the past dynasties, sand table models, imitation of the bronze acupuncture figure in the period of Guangxu of the Qing Dynasty, medical instruments of ethnic minorities, and medical books of the Ming Dynasty. The most treasured piece of the museum is the bronze acupuncture figure, which was made by Nanjing Museum, an imitated bronze figure from the imperial hospital during the reign of Emperor Guangxu in the Qing Dynasty. The bronze figure was transferred to the Palace Museum in 1925 and transferred to the Nanjing Museum in the spring of 1933 along with the third batch of cultural relics. In 1958, it was returned to the Museum of Chinese History. It is said that this bronze figure is a copy of Wiseman Bronze Figure by Wang Weiyi, a famous doctor in the Northern Song Dynasty. However, the vicissitudes of life changed so much that the two bronze figures cast by Wang Weiyi himself finally disappeared. It is recorded that bronze acupuncture figures were used in ancient times for teaching and examinations. The concrete approach is to coat the surface of the body with yellow wax, and then fill the body with water. When the student stabbed the acupoint correctly, water would flow out of the acupoint. If not, it means the student couldn't find the acupoint accurately. In this way, the teacher could accurately judge the learning situation of the students.

## 第二节　上海中医药博物馆
### Shanghai Museum of Traditional Chinese Medicine

　　上海中医药博物馆是全国中医药文化宣传教育基地，有80余年的历史，馆藏文物1万余件。馆外有1万平方米的百草园，种有600多种药用植物。镇馆之宝是摆放在二楼展厅的1744年铸造的针灸铜人。据文字记载，清代乾隆年间编纂了综合性医学丛书——《医宗金鉴》，这座针灸铜人是乾隆皇帝对编者的赏赐。而当时制作的这批针灸铜人如今国内仅存此一件了。博物馆还收藏有古代的医疗器具，如一套南北朝时期的手术器械、晋代的丹丸、宋代的黑釉大药罐、明代的香炉等，一件件文物诉说着中医药发展的千年历程。博物馆展厅设有多处模拟场景，如太医署多媒体场景，它演绎着我国唐朝由国家设立的医学院教学医疗的情况。针灸铜人的互动场景，它模拟着古人的针灸教学和考试的情况。脉象仪能让参与者感受到平时中医常说的滑脉、弦脉和洪脉。而四诊仪，通过多媒体的望闻问切能告诉参与者他的体质状况，指导他选择健康的生活方式。

　　With a history of more than 80 years, Shanghai Museum of Traditional Chinese Medicine is a national base for the promotion and education of TCM culture. It has a collection of more than

10,000 cultural relics. Outside, there is a garden of 10,000 square meters with more than 600 kinds of medicinal plants. The most treasured piece of the museum is a bronze acupuncture figure of 1744 in the exhibition hall on the second floor. According to written records, during the reign of Emperor Qianlong in the Qing Dynasty, a series of comprehensive medical books — *A Valuable Reference for Medicine* were compiled. At that time, a group of bronze acupuncture figures were presented as the gifts from Emperor Qianlong to the editors. But now, only one of them is remained in China. The museum also has collections of ancient medical instruments, such as a set of surgical instruments from the Northern and Southern Dynasties, a red pill from the Jin Dynasty, a large black-glazed medicine pot from the Song Dynasty, and a censer from the Ming Dynasty. Each piece of cultural relics tells the history of the development of TCM. The exhibition hall of the museum has several simulation scenes, such as the multi-media scene of the imperial medical department, which interprets the teaching of medicine established by the state during the Tang Dynasty. The interactive scene of bronze acupuncture figures, which simulates the teaching and examination of acupuncture of the ancients. The pulse apparatus allows participants to feel the smooth pulse, stringy pulse and full pulse commonly referred to in TCM. The four-diagnosis apparatus can tell the participant his physical condition and guide him to choose a healthy lifestyle through multimedia observation, listening and smelling, asking and pulse-taking.

## 第三节　藏医药文化博物馆
### Museum of Tibetan Medicine Culture

　　青海藏医药文化博物院是唯一一座集藏文化收藏、保护、展示、研究为一体的综合型博物馆。目前，馆藏文物达58000余件，内设16个大展厅。载入吉尼斯世界纪录的"镇馆之宝"《中国藏族文化艺术彩绘大观》长卷，画面绚丽多彩、气势恢宏，令人叹为观止。该长卷由当代藏族著名唐卡工艺美术大师宗者拉杰历时23年设计策划，由400余位藏、蒙、汉、土族顶尖工艺美术师耗时4年精心创作完成。卷长618米、宽2.5米，采用藏族传统绘画技艺，使用金粉、玉石、珊瑚等珍贵颜料精心绘制而成，其内容博大精深，包括藏族对宇宙形成的认识、历史、宗教、医学、文化生活等诸多方面，堪称藏族文化的百科全书。藏医药文化是藏族人民传统生活、传统人文精神和养身之道的物化表征，是青藏高原先民在本土医学经验基础上博采古印度医学、传统西方医学、传统中医学之长，通过藏医学各学派相互渗透、相互融合形成的。

　　Qinghai Tibetan Medicine Culture Museum is the only comprehensive museum that integrates cultural collection, protection, display and research. At present, the museum has a collection of more than 58,000 pieces of cultural relics and 16 exhibition halls. Ended in the Guinness World Records, the most treasured piece, the long volume of the *Chinese Tibetan Culture and Art Painting*

*Panorama*, is colorful, magnificent and breathtaking. Zongze Lajie, a well-known contemporary Tibetan master of Thangka arts and crafts, took 23 years to design and plan this long scroll and more than 400 top artists and crafts men from Tibetan, Mongolian, Han and Tu minorities spent 4 years in finishing the elaborate creation. With a length of 618 meters and a width of 2.5 meters, the scroll is elaborately painted with gold powder, jade, coral and other treasures in traditional Tibetan painting techniques. Its extensive and profound contents include Tibetan understanding of the formation of the universe, history, religion, medicine, cultural life and other aspects, which can be called the encyclopedia of Tibetan culture. The Tibetan medicine culture is the physical representation of the traditional life, traditional humanistic spirit and the way of health care of the Tibetan people. It was formed through the mutual penetration and integration of various schools of Tibetan medicine and drew upon the medical experience from the ancient Indian medicine, traditional western medicine and TCM.

## 第四节　国家图书馆之甲骨文
## National Library of China — Inscriptions on Oracle Bones

　　甲骨文是甲文和骨文的简称。甲文多刻在龟的腹甲上，骨文主要刻在牛胛骨和鹿头骨上，两者合称龟甲兽骨文字。甲骨文的发现与中医药有着不解之缘。清朝末年，一位名叫王懿荣的人是一位金石学家，他同时也爱好考古。1899年，王懿荣患痢疾，服用的药里有一味"龙骨"。他发现有些"龙骨"上面居然刻有与金文相似的文字，他就到处打听这种龙骨的来历，最终他得知是距河南安阳西北五里的小屯村农民卖给小药铺的，而此处原来是商代国都所在地。"龙骨"由此而成为发现甲骨文的重要契机，甲骨文从此被世人所重视。甲骨文的出土证明了商代的确存在过，以实物印证了中华三千多年的文明。有关资料显示，目前国内共藏有甲骨13万余片，现收藏在国家图书馆3.5万余片、故宫博物院2.2万余片、中国社科院考古所6600多片、山东博物馆4500多片，以及国内的各大博物馆。甲骨文中涉及疾病记载的有300余片，400余辞，记载了上百个病名（归纳为现代的34种疾病），是我国最早的医学档案。

　　Jiaguwen is the abbreviation for oracle-bone inscriptions. It is mostly carved on the tortoise's belly shells or on the cow scapula bones and the deer's skulls, which are collectively called inscriptions on tortoise shells or animal bones. The discovery of oracle-bone inscriptions is closely related to TCM. At the end of the Qing Dynasty, a man named Wang Yirong was an expert in epigraphy who also took interest in archaeology. In 1899, Wang Yirong suffered from dysentery and administered a prescription of Chinese medicines containing "dragon bone (tortoise shell)". He found some of them with similar inscriptions on them. He inquired about the origin of these shells and finally learned that they had been sold to a small pharmacy by some peasants in Xiaotun Village, 5 miles northwest of Anyang City of Henan Province, where the capital of the Shang Dynasty was originally located. The shells thus became an important opportunity for people to discover oracle-bone inscriptions, which was later taken seriously by the world. The unearthed oracle-bone inscriptions prove that the Shang Dynasty did exist and the Chinese civilization of more than three thousand years has been confirmed in real objects. At present, according to relevant data, there are more than 130,000 pieces of oracle bones in China, which are stored in the National Library of China (over 35,000 pieces), the Palace Museum (over 22,000 pieces), the Institute of Archaeology (over 6,600 pieces) of the Chinese Academy of Social Sciences, Shandong Museum (over 4,500 pieces) as well as other major museums in China. There are more than 300 bone pieces and over 400 sentences related to diseases recorded in the inscriptions, including hundreds of disease names (summarized as 34 diseases of modern times). It is the earliest medical archives in China.

# 第五节　故宫博物院之《清明上河图》
## The Palace Museum － *Riverside Scene at Qingming Festival*

　　《清明上河图》是我国十大传世名画之一，长528.7厘米，宽24.8厘米，现藏于北京故宫博物院，是北宋著名画家张择端唯一存世的一幅精品。关于作者的身世，千百年来一直是难解之谜。《清明上河图》在中国乃至世界绘画史上都是独一无二的。在5米多长的画卷里，绘有数量庞大的各色人物，各种牲畜，各种交通工具，以及各有特色的房屋、桥梁、城楼等，体现了宋代建筑的特征，具有很高的历史价值和艺术价值。《清明上河图》历来被视为研究北宋民俗生活、工商贸易、建筑形制、交通工具的重要史料。作者以写实的手法和精湛的画技再现了汴京的物阜民丰。北宋是社会稳定繁荣，医学大发展的时代，仔细端详画卷，也不难寻觅中医中药的踪迹。《清明上河图》绘有多处药铺和诊所，其中描绘最翔实的是画卷末端的"赵太丞家"。除此以外，《清明上河图》中还有刘家药店、杨家诊所及药摊等与医药相关的场景，可见医药与民众生活息息相关。北宋时期医药产业的繁荣和鲜明特色由此可见一斑。

　　*Riverside Scene at Qingming Festival* is one of China's top ten famous paintings. It is 528.7 cm long and 24.8 cm wide. It is the only outstanding painting by the famous painter Zhang Zeduan of the Northern Song Dynasty. His story has remained a mystery for thousands of years. *Riverside Scene at Qingming Festival* is unique in the history of painting in China and even in the world. In the five-meter-long scroll, there are a large number of different kinds of people, livestock and vehicle as well as architecture, reflecting the characteristics of the Northern Song Dynasty, which is of high historical and artistic value. *Riverside Scene at Qingming Festival* has always been regarded as an important historical data for the study of folk life, industry and commerce, architectural forms and means of transportation in the Northern Song Dynasty. The author reproduced the wealth of goods and people in Bianjing with a realistic technique and a rigorous painting technique. The Northern Song Dynasty was a time of social stability and prosperity and great development of medical science. It is not difficult to find traces of TCM, if you look carefully at the picture scroll. *Riverside Scene at Qingming Festival* depicts a number of pharmacies and clinics, among which the most detailed description is "Zhao Taicheng's Clinic" at the end of the scroll. In addition, in *Riverside Scene at Qingming Festival*, there are also scenes related to medicine, such as Liu's pharmacy, Yang's clinic and drug stall, which shows that medicine is closely related to people's life in the Northern Song Dynasty. The prosperity and distinctive characteristics of medicine industry in the Northern Song Dynasty can be seen from this.

# 药用植物园
## Medicinal Botanical Gardens

　　药用植物园是一个集中草药资源保存、研究、开发，以及科普、教育、文化宣传于一体的大型中医药现代科技园区，是药用植物保护区和药用植物开发利用技术中心。我国有药用植物1.1万余种，分布于各种不同的生态环境中，其中相当大一部分植物除有药用价值外，还具有极高的观赏价值。因此，按园林设计的要求，完全采用药用植物建设一个园林化的、具有中医药文化特点的药用植物园是可行的。用药用植物制作园林景观是中国园林艺术与中医药结合的产物，将成为我国园林艺术的一大特色，对世界园林园艺也将产生积极的影响。药用植物园的建立体现了中医药学丰富的文化内涵，向世界展示中国悠久的文化历史和各民族传统医药学，为人们创造了一个优美的自然环境。同时，由于药用植物在生长过程中不断释放出具有一定医药作用的化学物质，对人体有一定的保健作用，可作为自然疗法中的一种。品种繁多的药用植物的集中种植也为药用植物的生物多样性研究、资源开发与保护研究、药用植物的教学，提供了良好的环境和条件。

目前，国内已有北京药用植物园、广西药用植物园及贵阳药用植物园等十几处大型药用植物园。

Medicinal Botanical Gardens are large-scale modern scientific and technological parks of TCM, which focuses on the conservation, research and development of herbal medicine resources as well as scientific education and cultural propaganda. They are also the protection zones and the technical centers of the development and utilization of medicinal plants. There are over 11,000 species of medicinal plants in China, which are distributed in various ecological environments. A considerable part of them are of high ornamental value besides medicinal use. Therefore, according to the requirements of garden design, it is feasible to construct a medicinal botanical garden with the characteristics of TCM culture. The use of medicinal plants to make a garden landscape based on the combination of Chinese garden art and TCM will become one of the great artistic features of Chinese gardens and have a positive impact on the world gardening. The establishment of medicinal plant gardens reflects the rich cultural connotation of TCM, showing the long cultural history of China and the traditional medicine of various ethnic groups to the world and creating a beautiful natural environment for people. At the same time, due to the gradual release of medicinal effects in the process of botanical growth, the chemical substances may have a certain health care benefit to the human body and can be used as a natural therapy. The intensive cultivation of a wide variety of medicinal plants also provides a good environment and conditions for the study of the biodiversity of medicinal plants, the research of resource development and protection and the teaching of medicinal plants. At present, there are more than ten large medicinal botanical gardens in China, such as Beijing medicinal botanical garden, Guangxi medicinal botanical garden and Guiyang medicinal botanical garden, etc.

# 体验篇

PART II
EXPERIENCE

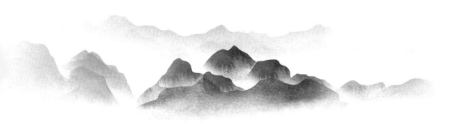

# 养生观
## Overview of Health Care

## 第一节 养生观概述
### Philosophy of Health Care

春秋战国时期，人文思潮兴起，中华养生学萌芽，先秦诸子著作中，几乎家家都有关于健身长寿的论述。后经华佗、董仲舒、嵇康、孙思邈、葛洪、陶弘景等人阐述和弘扬，特别是道家、儒家和医家文化的相互渗透，中华养生学终于形成了一套完整的体系。养生，原指道家通过各种方法颐养生命、增强体质、预防疾病，从而达到延年益寿的一种医事活动。养，即调养、保养、补养之意。生，即生命、生存、生长之意。现代意义的"养生"指的是根据人的生命规律主动进行物质与精神的身心养护活动。养生就是保养五脏，使生命得以绵长的意思。养生学是一门涉及诸多学科的综合科学，包括中医学、康复学、营养学、美学、心理学、国学、物理学、化学、艺术、烹饪、运动学、道学等。现代养生的含义是以中西医学理论为指导，用健康科学的图文、音乐、行为、活动、器械、饮食等，通过调节个人生活习惯、生活环境及心理状态，来调理身心，达到未病先防、消除不适、促愈已病、病后复原的保健目的。

During the Spring and Autumn Period and the Warring States Period, the humanistic trend of thought arose and the idea of health maintenance sprouted. In the works of the pre-Qin Dynasty, fitness and longevity were even household topics. Later, through the elaboration and promotion of Hua Tuo, Dong Zhongshu, Ji Kang, Sun Simiao, Ge Hong, Tao Hongjing and others, especially under the influence of Taoism, Confucianism and medical culture, Chinese health maintenance finally formed a set of complete system. Health preservation originally referred to a kind of medical activity that taoists used various methods to take care of life, enhance physical fitness and prevent diseases so as to prolong life. "Yang", means recuperation, maintenance and invigoration. "Sheng" is the meaning of life, including survival and growth. The modern meaning of "health preservation" refers to the active physical and mental activities according to the law of human life. Health preservation is to maintain the five zang-organs so that life can be long. Health maintenance is a comprehensive system involving many disciplines, including TCM, rehabilitation, nutriology, aesthetics, psychology, traditional Chinese culture, physics, chemistry, art, cuisine, kinematics, Taoism and so on. The meaning of modern health keeping is guided by the theories of Chinese and western medicine with pictures, texts, music, behavior, activities, equipment, diet, etc. Through the adjustment of personal living habits, living environment and psychological state, the body and mind is regulated to achieve the health purpose of prevention before the onset of disease, elimination of discomfort, promoting recovery and rehabilitation.

## 第二节 养生的种类
## Types of Health Care

养生是一种以中医为主、中西结合的科学养生体系，主要包括以下几类。（1）季节养生：按照春、夏、秋、冬的四季变化，调整饮食起居。春天养阳养肝，夏天养心健脾，秋天补肺润燥，冬天补气养阴。（2）时辰养生：中医认为人体五脏六腑在不同的时辰有不同的功能体现，人体的12条经络对应着12个时辰，如能顺应这规律来养护五脏六腑，我们就能远离疾病的困扰。（3）经络养生：根据中医经络原理，利用拔罐、刮痧、导引按跷、艾灸等方法，激发人体的自动调节和自我修复能力，以达到恢复健康的目的。（4）体质养生：根据不同的体质类型，采取不同的养生及食疗方法。（5）饮食养生：根据不同的体质及营养需要，在不同的时辰给予不同种类的营养摄入，以达到纠正体质偏差和平衡脏腑阴阳的目的，促进身体恢复健康。另外，还有运动养生、音乐养生等。

Health care is a kind of scientific system based on TCM with reference to contemporary medicine. Here we will introduce its types. (1) Seasonal health preservation: With natural changes of the four seasons, it is proper to adjust diet and pace of one's daily life, namely, nourishing yang and the liver in spring, nourishing the heart and invigorating the spleen in summer, nourishing the lung and moistening dryness in autumn, tonifying qi and nourishing yin in winter. (2) Time health preservation: according to TCM, the human organs function with time. The 12 meridians of the human body correspond to 24 hours. If we can comply with this law to maintain the five zang-organs and six fu-organs, we can stay away from the trouble of disease. (3) Meridian health preservation: According to the principle of TCM meridians, cupping, scraping, tuina and daoyin, moxibustion and other methods are applied to stimulate the body's automatic regulation and self-repair ability, thus achieving the purpose of restoring health. (4) Constitutional health preservation: Measures for health care are taken according to different types of physiques. (5) Dietary health preservation: according to different physiques and nutritional needs, different kinds of nutrition intake are given at different times in order to achieve the purpose of correcting the physique deviation and the imbalance of yin and yang of the viscera and promoting the body to restore health. In addition, there are other methods for health care, such as sports, music therapy, etc.

养生观 第四章

# 饮食养生
## Health Preservation with Food

## 第一节 药 酒
### Medicated Liquor

　　药酒在历代的医疗和养生保健实践中被证实确实有祛邪扶正、延年益寿的功效。李时珍在《本草纲目》中列举了69种不同功效的药酒，如五加皮酒、当归酒、人参酒、黄精酒、菊花酒、茯苓酒、桂花酒等，都是以白酒为原料的各种药酒。首先，酒的发散之性可以帮助药力外达于表，使理气行血药物的作用得到较好的发挥，也能使滋补药物补而不滞。其次，中药的多种成分能够溶于酒精，许多药物的有效成分可借助于酒的这一特性提取出来。此外，酒精还有防腐作用，能使中药材保存数月甚至数年而不变质。酒之所以受到古代医家的重视，一个重要原因就是适量饮酒具有养生保健作用。中国酒文化历史悠久，讲究饮酒方式便是其特点之一。酒在不冷不热时喝才是适宜的。饮酒应慢，不可速饮豪饮。饮酒需适度，太过损伤身体，不及等于起不到养生作用。酒在中医治疗中有着极为重要的地位和作用，酒本身是药食两得之品，很多药物因酒制而直达病灶，提高了疗效，因此药酒是人们乐于接受的一种养生形式。

Medicated liquor has been proved to have the effect of dispelling the pathogenic factors, strengthening the vital qi and prolonging life in the medical treatment and health care practice in successive dynasties. In *Compendium of Materia Medica*, Li Shizhen listed 69 kinds of medicated liquor with different effects, such as acanthopanax root bank liquor, angelica liquor, ginseng liquor, solomonseal rhizome liquor, chrysanthemum liquor, poria liquor, osmanthus liquor, etc., all of which were made with Chinese Baijiu. First, the dispersing effect of liquor can help the efficacy of drugs to reach the body surface so that the effect of regulating qi and blood drugs is improved and the tonic drugs function smoothly without stagnation. Second, a variety of components of Chinese medicine can be dissolved in alcohol and their active components can be extracted by virtue of this characteristic. In addition, alcohol has a preservative effect, keeping medicines from going bad for months or even years. The reason why liquor was recommended by doctors in ancient China is that it had the function of keeping in good health. China has a long history of liquor culture. One of its characteristics is the particular way of drinking it. A proper way will be beneficial to health if it is served at an appropriate temperature. Drinking should be done at a slow pace and swigging is improper. A moderate amount is good for health while excessive drinking is harmful to the body. Inadequate intake has no effect at all. Liquor plays a very important role in the treatment of TCM, as it is a product of both medicine and food. The effects can function quickly on the lesion due to the medicated liquor with the efficacy improved, so medicated liquor is a form of health care that is well received by people.

## 第二节　春节与酒
**The Spring Festival and Liquor**

　　有一种说法认为屠苏酒始于晋朝。据说有人住在草庵，每年除夕，将药囊丢到井中。到元日取水出来放在酒樽中，全家的人一起喝就不担心生病了。屠，就是割；苏，就是药草。砍了药草泡在井水中，泡成的水就是俗称"屠苏酒"。饮屠苏酒的习惯，是一家人中年纪最小的先喝，依次排下来，年纪越大的越后喝。原因是小孩过年增加了一岁，所以大家要祝贺他。而老年人过年则是生命又少了一岁，拖一点时间后喝，有祝他长寿的意思。另一种说法认为屠苏酒的配方出自华佗，又被孙思邈、李时珍等诸多名医推崇，无数典籍所传载，以及中国民间千百年口耳相传，久而久之，元日佳节饮屠苏酒便成了民风民俗。民间屠苏酒所用的药物是麻黄、川椒、细辛、防风、苍术、干姜、肉桂、桔梗。将它们各等分制成粗末，装入绢袋，浸入适量白酒中，密封3日后可饮用。屠苏酒可以祛风散寒，温中健脾，预防瘟疫。但饮用需适量。此配方对人体裨益甚多，可谓是兼滋补保健、防病疗疾、驱邪避瘴等多种功效的良方。

Saying has it that people started to take Tu Su liquor during the Jin Dynasty. Someone who lived in a thatched hut dropped bags of herbal medicine into the well every Eve of the Spring Festival. On the first day of the Spring Festival, he took water from the well and put it in the drinking vessels, so that the whole family could drink together and not be afraid of illness. "Tu" means cutting while "Su" means herbs. Cut down herbs and make the medicated beverage, thus getting the name of Tu Su. The service of drinking Tu Su liquor starts first from the youngest in the family, then goes down to the older in turn, finally, the oldest. The reason is that the child is growing up, so we should congratulate him. While the elderly loses another year of his life on earth after the Spring Festival. Delaying in service is to express the wish of a long life to him. Legend has it that the recipe of Tu Su liquor came from Hua Tuo and was highly praised by many famous masters such as Sun Simiao and Li Shizhen, etc., and that Tu Su liquor was recorded in many classic books and won public praise of Chinese folks. Over time, drinking Tu Su liquor on the first day of the Spring Festival has formed a folk custom. The drugs and methods used in the folk production of Tu Su liquor is to make equal amounts of Chinese ephedra, Sichuan pepper, asari radix, divaricate saposhnikovia root, atractylodes rhizome, dried ginger, cinnamon, balloonflower root into coarse powder. Put them into a silk bag, dip it into a moderate amount of Chinese Baijiu and seal the container. 3 days later, Tu Su liquor will be made. It can dispel wind and disperse cold, warm and invigorate the spleen and prevent plague, but you should drink it in moderation. This formula is very beneficial to the human body. Multiple functions include nourishing effect, health care, disease prevention and treatment and dispelling the pathogenic factors, etc.

## 第三节　端午节与酒
**Dragon Boat Festival and Liquor**

　　端午节在农历五月五日，人们为了辟邪、除恶、解毒，有饮菖蒲酒、雄黄酒的习俗。由于雄黄有毒，人们不再用雄黄兑制酒饮用了，只是在小孩面额上蘸雄黄酒写上个"王"字，以避邪祟，讨个健康成长的彩头。古人认为病从口入，多是邪杂之气，经口鼻吸入，于是把雄黄加水和酒洒于室内各个角落，认为可以辟邪、除恶。古人还在身上带着雄黄，不管走到哪里，都不用担心蛇害。雄黄虽然是中药，但并非植物，也不是动物制品，它是一种矿物。它有毒性，大多被当作外用药，但即便如此，大剂量或长时间使用，也会造成急性或慢性砷中毒。古人不懂化学毒性，虽然对于雄黄的使用很克制，但仍然存在风险。端午节饮雄黄酒是否有用，能防蛇吗？从科学的角度看，雄黄对蛇并没有特殊的作用和效果，更无法驱虫、安神、避秽。一般来说，没有经过医学训练，还是不要擅自饮用雄黄酒了，另外，如果处理不当，将雄黄加热，还会制造出"毒药"。因此，过端午节，吃粽子就可以了，雄黄酒能免则免吧。

On the fifth day of the fifth lunar month, Dragon Boat Festival, people have the custom of drinking calamus liquor or realgar liquor in order to ward off the pathogenic factors. Because realgar is poisonous, people no longer use it to make liquor. Instead, they just dip into realgar liquor and write the character " 王 " on children's forehead to avoid evil spirits and get a healthy growth. The ancients believed that diseases frequently came into the body from the mouth, so they mixed realgar with water and Chinese Baijiu together and then sprayed the liquid in every corner of the indoor, thinking this could avoid diseases. The ancients still carried realgar with them, no matter where they went, they did not have to worry about the harm of snakes. Realgar is a Chinese medicine, but it is not a plant or an animal product. It is a mineral. It is toxic and is mostly used externally, but even so, acute or chronic arsenic poisoning can occur in large doses or over a long period of time. The ancients did not understand chemical toxicity, although the use of realgar was very restrained, but there were still risks. Is it useful to drink realgar liquor? Can it protect against snakes? From a scientific point of view, realgar has no special effects on snakes, nor can it repel insects, calm spirits or avoid filth. Generally speaking, don't drink realgar liquor without medical consultation. In addition, if handled improperly, heating realgar liquor can be "poisonous". Therefore, it is proper and safe to eat Zongzi — rice wraped in bamboo leaves, on Dragon Boat Festival. The intake of realgar liquor should be abandoned.

## 第四节 重阳节与酒
**Double Ninth Festival and Liquor**

农历九月初九是重阳节。历代的中国人逢重九就要登高、赏菊、饮酒，此风俗延续至今。菊花酒，在古代被看作是重阳必饮、祛灾祈福的"吉祥酒"。因为九九与"久久"谐音，与"酒"也同音，因此派生出九九要喝菊花酒的说法。重阳节饮菊花酒是我国古代一个重要的节仪。无论宫中还是民间，都有重阳饮菊花酒一俗。菊花酒一般由菊花与糯米、酒曲酿制而成，古称"长寿酒"，其味清凉甜美，有养肝、明目、健脑、延缓衰老等功效。古代的文人墨客，也喜欢摘新鲜菊花泡酒饮，他们称这样的饮为"露饮"和"落英饮"。九月初九这天，采下初开的菊花和一点青翠的枝叶，掺和在准备酿酒的粮食中酿酒，待至第二年重阳饮用。古人认为，此酒能"祛百病，令长寿"。人们还在酒里面加入中草药，如加入地黄、当归、枸杞等中草药，健身效果更佳。除了饮菊花酒，有些人还饮茱萸酒、茱菊酒、黄花酒、薏苡酒、桑落酒、桂酒等。

The Double Ninth Festival falls on the ninth day of the ninth lunar month. The custom of climbing mountains, enjoying chrysanthemums and drinking medicated liquor on that day continues today. Chrysanthemum liquor, in ancient times, was regarded as the "auspicious liquor" to remove catastrophes during the Double Ninth Festival. Because the Chinese character "九" in double shares the same pronunciation with "久久" (longevity) and "酒" (liquor), it is derived from the saying of drinking chrysanthemum liquor that day. Moreover, drinking chrysanthemum liquor during the Double Ninth Festival was an important ritual in ancient China. Since ancient times, whether in the royal family or among folk people, there has been a custom of drinking chrysanthemum liquor on the day of the Double Ninth. Chrysanthemum liquor is generally made from chrysanthemum, glutinous rice and starter. It was called "longevity liquor" which tastes cool and sweet with functions of nourishing the liver, keeping eyes bright and brain healthy, anti-aging and other effects. In ancient times, some literati also liked to pick fresh chrysanthemums and drink liquor, which they called "dew drinking" and "falling flower drinking". On the ninth day of the ninth lunar month, the newly blossomed chrysanthemums and a few verdure branches and leaves are mixed with the grain to make liquor, which is to be drunken on the next Double Ninth Festival. The ancient believed that this liquor could dispel diseases and prolong life. People also added several Chinese herbs to the liquor for better fitness effects, such as rehmannia glutinis, Chinese angelica and wolfberry. In addition to the chrysanthemum liquor, some people also drank cornel liquor, zhuju liquor, yellow flower liquor, coix seed liquor, sangluo liquor and osmanthus liquor.

## 第五节 茶 药
### Medicated Tea

茶药是祖国传统医学中一个重要组成部分，它的历史非常悠久，历代医书中均有记载，最早记载茶药方剂的是三国时期张揖所著的《广雅》。茶药指含有茶叶的药方制剂。茶叶有很多功效，可以防治内外妇儿各科的很多病症，所以茶不但是药，而且还是万病之药。如姜茶可用于治痢疾，薄荷茶、槐叶茶用于清热，橘红茶用于止咳，莲心茶用于止晕，三仙茶用于消食，杞菊茶用于补肝等。茶能消食去腻，降火明目，宁心除烦，清暑解毒，生津止渴。现代药理分析认为，茶中含有的茶多酚具有很强的抗氧化性和生理活性，可清除人体自由基，可阻断亚硝酸胺等多种致癌物质在体内合成。它还能吸收放射性物质，有防辐射的作用，从而保护人们的皮肤。目前一些较为流行的成品茶药多用滤泡纸或布袋包装，用沸水冲泡数分钟即可饮用。它们不仅便于携带，而且色香味更接近于饮茶的本色。此外，还有通过药剂加工制成的块状或颗粒型速溶茶，饮用起来方便卫生，还易于药物的溶化吸收。

Medicated tea with a long history in China is an important part of TCM. It was recorded in the medical books of many dynasties. The earliest record of tea prescription is *Guang Ya* written by Zhang Yi in the Three Kingdoms Period. Medicated Tea refers to prescriptions containing tea-leaves. As we know, tea has the effects of preventing and treating diseases related to gynecology, pediatrics, internal medicine and surgery, etc., so tea is not only used as a medicated material, but also used with a variety of herbs. For example, ginger tea is used to cure dysentery. Mint tea and pagoda leaf tea is used to clear away heat. Tangerine tea is used to stop cough. Lotus seed heart tea is used to stop halo. Sanxian tea is used to eliminate food retention. Chinese wolfberry and chrysanthemum tea is used to replenish the liver and so on. Tea can help dissolve greasy food, decrease internal heat, keep eyes bright, calm down the mind, detoxify, produce body fluid and quench thirst. Science has proved that tea contains polyphenols, which is a strong antioxidant to promote physiological activities. It is the scavenger of human free radicals and can block the synthesis of various carcinogens such as nitrite amine in the body. It can also absorb radioactive material to achieve the effect of avoiding radiation, thus protecting people's skin. At present, some of the more popular products are usually packaged in filter paper or cloth bag, and brewed with boiling water for a few minutes before drinking. This process, together with their color and aroma, is closer to the essence of drinking tea. In addition, the lumpy or granular instant tea is more convenient to drink up and the melted drug is also easy to be absorbed through the pharmaceutical processing.

## 第六节 药 粥
## Medicated Porridge

粥，俗称稀饭。中国人有食粥的习惯，而且花色品种特别多。冬夏季节不同，粥的功用也各异。尤其是早餐，老人们还是习惯喝粥。喝牛奶、豆浆，用他们的话说就跟没吃一样，还是来碗粥喝着舒服。从古至今，粥的品种越来越多，有大米粥、小米粥、八宝粥、紫米粥、绿豆粥、赤小豆粥、玉米粥等。此外，还有在粥里加进一些药食两用的药粥，如山药粥、南瓜粥、核桃粥、桂圆粥、枸杞粥、莲子芡实薏米粥等。人们可以根据自己不同的体质来食用不同的药粥。药粥之中毕竟含有药物成分，这就决定了药粥不能像普通的粥那样随意被食用，而必须要讲究对证原则，不可盲目食用。根据药粥中所添加药物的不同，其性质及治疗的病症也有所不同，一般而言，脾胃虚寒的人，应该食用有清补功效的药粥，如红枣粥、核桃粥等；阴虚内热的人，则宜服用绿豆粥、百合粥等。切不可随意服用，否则不仅起不到食疗的作用，还可能适得其反，损害健康。

Porridge, commonly known as gruel, has been a kind of staple diet for Chinese people and there are a lot of varieties. The function of porridge varies from season to season. Especially for breakfast, the old people still are used to taking it. Milk and soymilk, as they say, are not adequate for a breakfast. They think only a bowl of porridge will soothe the stomach. Since ancient times, there have been more and more varieties of porridge, which are made with rice, millet, eight-treasured rice, purple rice, mung beans, red beans, polenta and so on. In addition, there are some materials of both dietary and medicated properties mixed in the porridge, called medicated porridge, such as Chinese yam porridge, pumpkin porridge, walnut porridge, longan pulp porridge, Chinese wolfberry porridge, porridge of lotus seed, gordon eurale seed and coix seed, which are too many to enumerate. People can eat different kinds of medicated porridge according to their different constitutions. After all, a medicated porridge contains medicinal ingredients, which determines that it cannot be eaten at will like an ordinary porridge. Porridge should be served based on syndrome differentiation. Do not have it blindly. The nature of the porridge and the syndrome it treats vary from the drugs added. Generally speaking, those with deficient cold in the spleen and stomach are recommended to have the medicated porridge with mild nourishing effect, such as jujube porridge and walnut porridge, etc. It is appropriate for those with yin deficiency and heat in the interior to have mung bean porridge or lily bulb porridge. Be sure not to take it at will, otherwise it will not play the role of dietary therapy, which may be counterproductive and do damage to health.

# 第七节 花　膳
## Flower Cuisine

　　花膳是指以花卉为食材烹调而成的菜肴，由于花卉形、色、香、味俱佳的特点，花膳自然比一般菜肴更加赏心悦目、开胃可口，而且多了一番清雅情趣。如用韭菜花加盐制成糊状的佐料，是北京人吃火锅的必备之品。洋槐花甘甜清香，有清热凉血、行气解郁、和血止痛的功效，将洋槐花洗净加入面粉和油、盐等调味料拌匀，入笼屉蒸熟，是陕北民间常见的花膳。菊花有疏风散热、明目解毒之功，在广东地区有很多菜肴都以其为原料，如菊花炒肉片、菊花熘鱼片、菊花鱼丸等。云南地区的植物资源十分丰富，人们喜食的花卉就有100多种。著名的云南特色小吃鲜花饼就是以玫瑰花为主要原料制成的。现代科学家对花卉的化学成分进行了分析，花卉含有16～22种氨基酸及丰富的蛋白质、淀粉、脂肪，并含有维生素A、B、C以及铁、镁、钾、锌等微量元素，还含有抗菌和抗病毒成分。花卉具有一定的药用和保健功效。总之，花膳不但风味独特，更有一定保健作用。

Floral cuisines refer to dishes made by cooking with flowers. Due to the excellent shape, color, fragrance and taste of flowers, floral cuisines are naturally more pleasing to the eye, appetizing, and elegant than ordinary ones. For example, use leek flowers and salt to make a paste seasoning, which is an essential ingredient of Beijingers to have hot pot. Acacia flowers are sweet and fragrant, which can clear away heat, cool blood, activate qi and relieve depression and pain. Wash Acacia flowers, add flour, oil, salt and other seasonings, mix them well and then steam them. This is a common folk flower cuisine in northern Shaanxi. Chrysanthemum has the function of dissipating wind and cooling heat, improving eyesight and detoxification. In Guangdong, there are many dishes based on it, such as fried meat slices with chrysanthemum, fish slices with chrysanthemum, fish balls with chrysanthemum, etc.Yunnan region is very rich in plant resources. There are more than 100 kinds of flowers that people like to eat. The famous Yunnan specialty snack— flower cakes, are made with rose as the main raw material. Modern scientists have analyzed the chemical composition of flowers, which contain 16−22 kinds of amino acids, rich protein, starch, fat, vitamin A, B, C, iron, magnesium, potassium, zinc and other trace elements, as well as antibacterial and antiviral substances. Flowers have certain medicinal, health care functions and can enhance your physiques and prolong life. In a word a flower meal not only has unique flavor, but also can strengthen health.

## 第八节　五辛盘
### Five Spicy Vegetables

古人立春有吃"五辛盘"的习俗。除取其象征性的吉利意义之外，它还包含有一定的科学道理。立春之后，阴消阳长，休眠了一个冬天的植物开始萌发，人体也需要舒展。聪明的祖先选择食用辛味食物，帮助人体运行气血、发散邪气。这对于养阳、调动机体正气、保证机体健康和季节性防疫，都有积极的作用。药食同源存在使得民间对辛味药物或食物的运用积累了许多经验。民谚"冬吃萝卜夏吃姜，不劳医生开药方"就是辛味防病治病的经验写照。此外，用葱头熨肚脐、生姜熬汤、薄荷泡茶防治各种感冒、用烧酒或辣椒汤驱逐寒气、用红花酒活血行血等，也都是民间对辛味的具体运用。它们充分体现了中医药知识深厚的群众基础。春盘的内容并不十分严格，民间也有用葱、蒜、椒、姜、芥丝之类寻常菜蔬的，但总归是辛味食物。随着时间的推移，吃五辛盘成了一种习俗，这种习俗在各地也逐渐发生了变化。在北京，甚至变成了吃"春饼"，但其象征的意义是一样的。

The ancients had the custom of eating "five spicy vegetables" during the days of Beginning of Spring. In addition to its symbolic auspicious significance, there are also some scientific reasons. After Beginning of Spring, yin fades and yang grows. Plants that have lain dormant all winter begin to germinate and the human body needs to stretch as much as it likes. Wise ancestors chose spicy food to regulate qi and blood thus to eliminate the pathogenic factors, replenish yang, mobilize the body's vital energy and ensure the body's health and seasonal epidemic prevention. Due to the homologous relationship between medicine and food, many Chinese medicines are common food at the same time, so a lot of experience has also been created and accumulated in the folk use of spicy medicine or food. The popular saying "eat turnip in winter, ginger in summer and you don't have to visit a doctor" is the embodiment of preventing and treating diseases with spicy medicines or food. In addition, onion mashed to warm navel, ginger boiled into soup, mint made into tea to prevent various colds, Chinese liquor and pepper soup to repel the chill, safflower liquor to promote blood circulation, etc., are also the specific use of spicy flavor among folk people. They fully embody the folk wisdom of Chinese medicine. The content of a spring plate is not restricted to green onion, garlic, pepper, ginger, leaf mustard but other vegetables are commonly seen. As time went on, the custom of eating five spicy vegetables has gradually varied in different places. In Beijing, it has been evolved into "spring pancakes", but the symbolic meaning has not changed yet.

## 第九节　艾草美食
## Food with Mugwort

　　艾草是一味常见的中草药，因它对我们的健康有益，所以深受人们的喜爱。它有祛湿、止血、消炎以及平喘等功效。艾草也是一种很好的食物，具有一定的营养价值。艾草的吃法很多，我们可以用艾草搭配其他食材做成各种点心和菜肴。比如用它来包饺子，用它来煎鸡蛋，还可以用它来制作汤水或炖汤。在中国南方传统食品中，有一种糍粑就是用艾草作为主要原料做成的，用清明前后，将鲜嫩的艾草和糯米粉按一比二的比例和在一起，包上花生、芝麻及白糖等馅料，部分地区会加上绿豆蓉，再将它们蒸熟即可。在广东东江流域，当地人在冬季和春季采摘鲜嫩的艾草叶子和芽，作蔬菜食用。每逢立春时分赣州客家人有采集艾草做成艾米果的习俗。艾米果的形状与饺子有点像，但体积更大，里面包有馅料，可当作主食。艾草还可以被制作成"艾叶茶""艾叶汤""艾叶粥"等食物，食用这些食物可以增强人体对疾病的抵抗能力。你也可以尝试一下艾草做的馒头，含有天然色素的馒头，听起来就非常健康。

Mugwort is a common Chinese herbal medicine. It is good for our health, so it is popular with people. It has effects of clearing dampness, hemostasis, anti-inflammation and anti-asthma. Mugwort is also a good food with nutritional value. There are many ways to eat mugwort. We can use mugwort with other ingredients to make various snacks and dishes, such as dumplings, fried eggs and soups or stews. Among the traditional foods in the south of China, one kind of glutinous rice cake is made with mugwort as the main material. That is, peanut, sesame and sugar fillings are wrapped by the dough which is made by mixing the fresh mugwort grown during the Qingming Day and glutinous rice flour at a ratio of one to two. In some areas, mashed mung beans are added and steamed. Around the Dongjiang River in Guangdong Province, local people pick fresh wormwood leaves and buds in winter and spring to eat as vegetables. During the Beginning of Spring, the Hakka in Ganzhou have the custom of collecting mugwort to make mugwort rice cakes whose shape are similar to dumplings, but larger in size. They are also stuffed with fillings and can be used as a staple food. Mugwort can also be made into "mugwort tea" "mugwort soup" "mugwort porridge" and other recipes. Eating these foods can enhance the body's resistance to disease. You can also try steamed bread made with mugwort. Steamed bread with natural coloring looks very healthy.

# 起居养生
# Health Preservation in Daily Life

## 第一节 药 浴
## Medicated Bath

药浴是沐浴疗法中与中医学联系最密切的，属于中医外治法。用加有药物的水进行洗浴，具有疏通经络，活血化瘀，祛风散寒，清热解毒，消肿止痛等功效，又能使肌肤光滑润泽。一些散发芳香气味的药物能除湿辟秽，其优雅的香气还能增加沐浴的乐趣。药浴选用的药物根据季节和体质不同有所变化，最为人熟知的就是端午节药浴。它是预防疾病的有效方法，也成为民间的一种攘除灾疫、祈福求祥的仪式。端午节用于药浴的中草药很多，有兰草、艾叶、菖蒲、桑叶、薄荷、野菊花等等。除了汉族中草药药浴外，其他民族也有不同的药浴疗法。 藏医经典著作中提到将西藏传统的水浴、药浴、熏浴、蒸气浴、日光浴合称为"健康五浴"，并详述了操作方法。藏药浴采用藏区道地药材，具有祛痰化湿，清热解毒，活血化瘀，益肾壮腰等功效。另一种叫温泉浴的沐浴方式与药浴相似，只是它与自然环境联系密切，其要旨恐怕不止是清洁，更多的是舒缓身心，亲近自然。

Medicated bath, a therapy most closely related with TCM, belongs to the external treatment of TCM. The bath with medicated water can dredge the meridians, activate blood, remove stasis, dispel wind and cold, clear away heat and detoxify, relieve swelling and pain and make skin smooth and moist. Some sweet-smelling drugs can dehumidify and sweeten the bath with their elegant aroma. Drugs for bath differ according to seasons and individuals. The most familiar is the medicated bath during Dragon Boat Festival. It has become an effective way to prevent diseases as well as a folk ritual to avoid epidemic and pray for good luck. There are many Chinese herbs used for medicated bath in Dragon Boat Festival, such as eupatorium, mugwort, calamus, mulberry leaf, mint, wild chrysanthemum and so on. In addition to the herbal bath among Han people, other nationalities also have different ones. The classic works of Tibetan medicine recorded "five health baths", namely, the traditional Tibetan water bath, medicated bath, fumigation bath, steam bath and sunbath. The operative methods are explained in detail in the classic. Tibetan medicated bath adopts Tibetan genuine herbs, which has the functions of eliminating phlegm and dampness, clearing away heat and detoxification, promoting blood circulation and removing blood stasis, benefiting the kidney and strengthening the waist. Another form of bathing, called warm spring bath, is similar to a medicated bath, except that it is closely related to the natural environment and its main purpose may not only clean, but also soothe the body and mind and get close to nature.

# 第二节　药　枕
## Medicated Pillows

　　药枕是改善睡眠的一件生活好物。药枕中的药物多具有芳香走窜的性质，作用于头部的穴位，再通过经络的传导，对人体有调和气血、祛病延年的作用。药枕多适用于慢性疾病患者，如鼻炎、颈椎病、偏头痛、高血压等。用来充当枕芯的药物，通常选用质地轻柔的花、叶、籽类药物，不可过硬。如果使用质地较硬的药物，注意要将其研为粗末后再装入枕头，枕巾最好选用纯棉材质。松软的枕头不但枕起来舒适，而且还可增加头与枕之间的接触面积，使药物充分渗透到头颈部。药枕中的药物也有保质期，在不使用药枕时，为防止有效成分挥发，应当用塑料袋包好，一般2年就需更换一次枕内药物。药物过敏者和孕妇慎用药枕。民间常用荞麦皮、决明子、芦花等制成枕头，原料虽不及医书中品类繁多，但也有不错的养生防病效果。自己不妨尝试做一个药枕，把菊花、夏枯草各50克，研为粗末，装入布袋中当枕芯。

　　A medicinal pillow is helpful for good sleeping. Medicated pillows have the characteristic of aroma, which can harmonize qi and blood, dispel diseases and prolong life by acting on the acupuncture points in the head and the conduction of the meridian. Medicated pillows are more suitable for patients with chronic diseases, such as rhinitis, cervical spondylosis, migraine and hypertension, etc. The drugs used as pillow contents are usually soft and dried flowers, leaves and seeds. If you use a hard substance, grind it into a coarse powder before putting it into the pillow and the pillow towel is best made of pure cotton. Soft pillows are not only comfortable, but also can increase the contact area between the head and the pillow, allowing sufficient penetration of the herbs into your head and neck. Drugs in the pillow also have a shelf life. When the pillow is not used, it should be wrapped in plastic bags in order to prevent the active ingredients from volatilizing. Generally, the herbs in the pillow should be replaced every 2 years. Use with caution in people with drug allergies and pregnant women. Buckwheat husk, cassia seed and reed flowers are commonly used to make pillows. The materials, though less varied than those found in medical books, have good preventive effects for health. You might as well try making one with chrysanthemum, bugle each 50 grams ground to coarse granules and put into a cloth bag.

## 第三节　艾草、菖蒲
# Mugwort and Calamus

端午节是入夏后第一个节日，气温上升，正是疾病多发的时期，人们往往会在家门口、厅堂中挂几株艾草或菖蒲，形似利剑来驱病、防蚊、辟邪。挂艾草、菖蒲是汉族民间端午节的习俗。艾草是一种菊科多年生草本植物，它性温，味苦。艾的茎、叶都含有挥发性芳香油，能产生奇特的芳香，可驱蚊蝇、虫蚁，净化空气。中医学上以艾入药，有理气血、暖子宫、祛寒湿的功效。将艾叶加工成"艾绒"是灸法治病的重要药材。菖蒲是一种多年水生草本植物。它狭长的叶片也含有挥发性芳香油，是提神通窍、健骨消滞、杀虫灭菌的药物。挂艾草和菖蒲是有一定防病作用的。端午节除了挂艾枝，悬菖蒲，人们还洒扫庭院，洒雄黄水，饮雄黄酒，驱逐污浊和腐败之气，杀菌防病，因而这一天也是自古相传的"卫生节"。每个地方悬挂的习俗不一样，有单独挂艾草或菖蒲的。常见的做法是将艾草和菖蒲用红绳绑在一起，然后倒挂或者悬于门两边，代表驱走所有灾祸，保佑一家人平平安安。

Dragon Boat Festival is the first festival in summer. When the temperature rises, it is a period when diseases occur frequently. People often hang several plants of mugwort or calamus in their doorways and halls, which look like a sharp sword to drive away diseases, mosquitoes and evil. Hanging moxa leaves and calamus is a folk Dragon Boat Festival custom of the Han nationality. Mugwort is a perennial herb in the composite family with warm nature and bitter flavor. The stems and leaves of mugwort contain volatile aromatic oil, which can produce a peculiar aroma, repel mosquitoes, insects and ants, and purify air. In TCM, mugwort can be used as medicine, which may regulate qi and blood, warm uterus and dispel cold and dampness. "Moxa wool" processed from mugwort leaves is an important medicinal material for moxibustion. Calamus is a perennial aquatic herb. Its long and narrow leaves also contain volatile aromatic oil, which is a refreshing, bone-benifiting, anti-stagnation, insecticidal and sterilization drug. It is really effective in preventing diseases to hang mugwort leaves and calamus. In addition to hanging mugwort branches and calamus, people also sweep the courtyard, sprinkle realgar water, drink realgar liquor and drive away the dirty things for sterilization and disease prevention, thus this day has been called "Health Day" since ancient times. The hanging customs differ from place to place, singularly or together. A common practice is to tie mugwort and calamus together with red ropes, and then hang them upside down or on either side of the door in order to drive away all disasters and keep the whole family safe.

# 第四节　香　囊
## Sachets

香囊辟疫的方法被称为"香佩法"或"香嗅法"，是中医外治法的一种，即不通过内服药物，而是将药物或非药物施于皮肤、孔窍、俞穴及病变的局部来调整机体、疏通经络、沟通表里的一种养生方法。香佩法的施药方式一般有"佩、戴、着"三种。香佩法多用于预防传染病。香嗅法是指在香囊中放入不同的药物，通过口、鼻进入人体以期发挥辟邪气、扶正、解表、清气、祛湿、开窍等不同功效的方法。佩戴香囊可用来防治感冒、咳嗽、胸闷、心痛、眩晕、失眠、鼻塞、驱蚊等。有些中医院也会应用香囊给药预防荨麻疹或治疗带状疱疹。中药香囊治疗失眠症时会选用冰片、肉桂、朱砂等。预防腹泻时会选用肉桂、艾叶、苍术、白豆蔻、小茴香等。治疗慢性鼻炎会选用辛夷、薄荷、苍耳子。驱蚊可选用丁香、薄荷、薰衣草、陈皮、七里香或艾叶等。还有医师会配制香囊治疗高血压、心脏病、气管炎、慢性中耳炎、目赤肿痛等。平时若想增强免疫力，可选取丁香、紫苏、苍术、细辛等。

The method of preventing epidemic with sachets is called "wearing method" or "smelling method", which is a kind of TCM external treatment, meaning that the drug is not taken internally, but applied to the skin, pores, shu points and local lesions to adjust the body, dredge the meridians and connect the exterior and interior of man. There are three places of applying the sachet: the neck, waist, or skin. These methods are mostly used to prevent infectious diseases. And the method of smelling is to put different drugs in the perfume sac, sending fragrances through the mouth, nose into the human body in order to play the role of dispelling the pathogenic factors, strengthening the vital qi, relieving the exterior syndromes, clearing away dampness and other different effects. Wearing sachets of herbal medicine can be used to prevent and cure cold, cough, chest tightness, heartache, dizziness, insomnia, nasal congestion and drive mosquitoes. Some TCM hospitals also use sachets to prescribe for patients to prevent urticaria or treat herpes zoster. Sachets of herbal medicine will be used to treat insomnia with borneol, cinnamon and cinnabar, etc. For the prevention of diarrhea, cinnamon, mugwort, atractylodes, cardamom and fennel will be used. Chronic rhinitis can be treated with magnolia flower, mint and cocklebur fruit. Cloves, mint, lavender, tangerine peel, qilixiang or mugwort leaves, etc. can be chosen for mosquito repellents. Some doctors will prepare sachets to treat hypertension, heart disease, bronchitis, chronic otitis media, eye swelling and pain. Usually if you want to enhance immunity, you can choose clove leaf, perilla, atractylodes, asarum and other medicinal materials.

# 运动养生
## Exercise Regimen

## 第一节　养生十三法（一）
### Sun Simiao's 13 Ways to Keep Healthy (1)

　　孙思邈（581－682年），京兆华原（今陕西省铜川市）人，唐代医药学家。据说孙思邈幼时体弱多病，他便立志学医。他发明了养生十三法，并经常用此法锻炼。做法如下：（1）发常梳。将手掌互搓36下，掌心发热，然后由前额开始用手指梳理上去，经后脑梳至颈部。早晚做10次。经常做这动作，可以明目祛风，防止头痛、耳鸣、白发和脱发。（2）目常运。合眼，然后用力睁开眼，眼珠打圈，望向左、上、右、下四方。重复3次。接下来，搓手36下，将发热的掌心敷上眼部。这动作可以缓解眼睛疲劳，纠正近视。（3）齿常叩。口微微合上，上下排牙齿互叩，无须太用力，但牙齿互叩时须发出声响。轻轻松松慢慢做36下。这动作可以通上下颚经络，帮助保持头脑清醒，加强肠胃吸收、防止蛀牙和牙骨退化。（4）漱玉津。口微微合上，将舌头伸出牙齿外，由上面开始，向左慢慢转动，一共转

12圈，然后将口水吞下去。之后反方向再做一下。从现代科学角度分析，口水含有大量酵素，经常做这动作，可以强健肠胃，延年益寿。

Sun Simiao (581A.D. — 682A.D.) was born in Huayuan, Jingzhao (now Tongchuan City, Shaanxi Province). He was a medical expert and pharmacist in the Tang Dynasty. It is said that when Sun Simiao was young, he decided to study medicine due to his poor health. He invented the thirteen ways of keeping fit and often exercised with them. Here are steps to do them: (1) Comb your hair regularly. Rub palms together for 36 times until the palms get warm. Then start combing with your fingers from the forehead to the back of your head and neck. Do it 10 times respectively in the morning and evening. Doing this action often can dispel wind to make your eyes clear and prevent headache, tinnitus, white hair and hair loss. (2) Move your eyes often. Close your eyes and open them forcefully. Turn your eyes around and look to the left, up, to the right and down. Repeat them 3 times. Next, rub your hands 36 times and apply the warm palms to your eyes. This action can relieve eyestrain and correct myopia. (3) Frequent tooth knocking. Close your mouth slightly and tap the upper and lower rows of teeth against each other without too much force, but with a sound. Do it 36 reps slowly and easily. This action can clear the meridians around your mouth, help keep the mind clear, strengthen gastrointestinal absorption and prevent tooth decay and bone degeneration. (4) Swallow your saliva. Stick your tongue out of your teeth, starting at the top, slowly turning to the left, making 12 turns and then swallow the saliva. And then do it in the opposite direction. In modern science, saliva contains a lot of enzyme. Doing this action often can strengthen the stomach and prolong life.

## 第二节　养生十三法（二）
### Sun Simiao's 13 Ways to Keep Healthy (2)

（5）耳常鼓。用手掌掩住双耳，用力向内压，然后放手，应该有"卜"的一声。重复做10下。双掌掩耳，将耳朵反折，双手食指压住中指，以食指用力弹后脑风池穴10下，卜卜有声。这动作每天临睡前做，可以增强记忆和听觉。（6）面常洗。搓手36下，暖手以后上下扫面或向外在面部画圈。经常做这动作，可以令脸色红润有光泽，同时不会有皱纹。（7）头常摇。双手叉腰，闭目，垂下头，缓缓向右扭动，直至恢复原位为一次，共做6次。反方向重复。经常做这动作可以令头脑灵活，防止颈椎增生。不过，注意要慢慢做，否则会头晕。（8）腰常摆。身体和双手有韵律地摆动。当身体扭向左时，右手在前，左手在后，在前的右手轻轻拍打小腹，在后的左手轻轻拍打"命门"穴位。反方向重复。至少做50下，做够100下更好。这动作可以强化肠胃、固肾气，防止消化不良、胃痛、腰痛。（9）腹常揉。搓手36下，手暖后两手交叉，围绕肚脐顺时针方向揉36下。这动作可以帮助消化吸收、消除腹部鼓胀。

(5) Pat the back of your head often. Cover your ears with your palms and press them inward. Then let go. There should be a peep. Repeat this for 10 times. Then cover your ears with your palms, fold

your ears back and press your middle fingers with your index fingers. Beat fengchi acupoint 10 times with your forefingers adequately. Do this every night just before you go to bed. It may improve your memory and hearing. (6) Rub your face regularly. Rub your hands 36 times, then warm your face up and down or outward. Doing this action often can give your face a ruddy luster and the wrinkles may fade away. (7) Shake your head slightly. Put your hands on hips with your eyes closed and head down. Slowly twist your head to the right until back to the original position. Do it 6 times in total. Repeat it in the opposite direction. Doing this regularly can keep your mind flexible and prevent cervical hyperplasia. Do it slowly, though, or you'll get dizzy. (8) Always swing your waist. Move your body and hands in rhythm. When the body twists to the left, the right hand is in front and the left hand behind. Gently pat the lower abdomen with the right hand in front and the life gate point with the left hand in the back. Repeat it in the opposite direction. Do it at least 50 times and even better for 100 times. This action can strengthen the stomach and kidney and prevent indigestion, stomachache and pain in your low back. (9) Rub your belly often. Rub your hands 36 times. After your hands are warm, cross your hands and knead clockwise around your navel 36 times. This will help digestion and absorption and eliminate abdominal distension.

## 第三节　养生十三法（三）
**Sun Simiao's 13 Ways to Keep Healthy (3)**

（10）摄谷道，即提肛。吸气时提肛，即将肛门的肌肉收紧。屏住呼吸，维持数秒，直至不能忍受，然后呼气放松。这动作无论何时都可以练习。最好是每天早晚各做20下至30下。相传这动作是十全老人乾隆最得意的养生功法。（11）膝常扭。双脚并排，膝部紧贴，人微微下蹲，双手按膝，向左右扭动，各做20下。这动作可以强化膝盖关节，所谓"人老腿先老、肾亏膝先软"。要延年益寿，得从双脚做起。（12）常散步。挺直胸膛，轻松地散步。最好心无杂念，尽情欣赏沿途景色。民间有个说法，"饭后走一走，活到九十九"。虽然有点夸张，不过，散步确实是有益的运动。（13）脚常搓。右手搓左脚，左手搓右脚。由脚跟至脚趾，再搓回脚跟为一下。共做36下。接下来两手大拇指轮流搓脚心涌泉穴，共做100下。常做这动作，可以治失眠、降血压、消除头痛。脚底集中了全身器官的反射区。经常搓脚可以强化各器官，对身体有益。上述介绍的孙思邈养生十三法，虽然简单，但可以帮助我们达到养生的目的。

(10) Contract the anus. When inhaling, tighten the muscles of the anus. Hold your breath for a few seconds until you can't stand it, then exhale to relax. This can be practiced at any time. It's best

to do 20 to 30 repetitions each morning and evening. Legend has it that this was the Emperor Qianlong of the Qing Dynasty's favorite regimen. (11) Turn your knees. Stand with your feet side by side and your knees close together. Squat slightly with your hands on your knees and twist to the left and right. Do it 20 times each. This action can strengthen your knee joint, which avoids the so-called "weakness of your knees precedes weakness of your kidneys". To be healthy, start with movement of your feet. (12) Take regular walks. Straighten your chest and take a brisk walk. Best of all, enjoy the scenery along the way. There is a folk saying, "Walk after dinner and you'll live to ninety-nine." It's a bit of an exaggeration, but walking is a good exercise. (13) Rub your feet often. Rub your left foot with your right hand and your right foot with your left. Rub from heel to toe and then back to heel. Do 36 reps. Next use two thumbs to take turns to wipe yongquan point for a total of 100. This action can help treat insomnia, hypertension and headache. The soles of the feet have the reflection zones of the organs. Rubbing your feet regularly strengthens your organs and is good for your body. The thirteen regimens of Sun Simiao introduced above are simple, but they can help us achieve the goal of health preservation.

## 第四节 太极拳
### Taijiquan

太极拳与养生息息相关，它的养生思想主要来源于儒家、道家和中医养生等方面，其机理主要体现在调和气血、平衡阴阳、疏通经络、调节脏腑等方面。太极拳基于太极阴阳的理念，用意念统领全身，通过入静放松、以意导气、以气催形的反复习练，来达到修身养性、陶冶情操、强身健体、益寿延年的目的。太极拳的套路有多种多样，其架势大小不同，重心高低不同，动作快慢也不同。习练者可根据自身不同的体质，选择适合的套路。但不论何种套路的太极拳，其动作都要求发于意，松而有力地交替转化，即所谓的柔中有刚。练起拳来随一吸一呼，动作一开一合，缓缓地连绵不断。而且，锻炼并非一朝一夕的事，要经常习练。习练太极拳不仅是对身体的锻炼，也是对意志和毅力的锻炼。适当的打太极拳可以调摄保养人体，提高人体的正气以抵抗外邪。长期坚持锻炼不仅可以预防疾病，还可治疗多种疾病。

Taijiquan is closely related to health preservation whose thoughts mainly came from Confucianism, Taoism and TCM health preservation. Its mechanism is mainly embodied in harmonizing qi and blood, balancing yin and yang, dredging the meridians, regulating viscera and so on. This concept, based on yin and yang of taiji, enables the exersicer to command his whole body with his mind. Through the repeated practice of relaxation into meditation, guiding qi by his mind and exersicing by qi, the exerciser achieves the purpose of cultivating and strengthening his body and mind, thus achieving a state of prolonging life. There are various sets of taijiquan with different frames, gravity centers and movement paces. The trainee can choose the proper set according to his or her constitution. But no matter which set, its movements are required to be done in an intentional, loose and powerful alternations, which is so-called "softness comes with strength". When you practice taijiquan, your movements open and close as you breathe in and out, slowly and continuously. What's more, exercise should be done regularly and continuously. Practicing taijiquan is not only a physical exercise, but also an exercise of will and perseverance. Proper taijiquan exercise can regulate and maintain the human body and improve its ability to resist the exopathogenic factors. Exercise over a long period of time not only prevents but also cures many diseases.

# 治疗养生
## Treatment and Rahabilitation

## 第一节 煎 药
### Decoct Chinese Medicine

煎药，是指将中药放入锅中进行煎煮的一种方式。煎药前，先把中药用冷水泡30分钟以上，水要淹没药面，高出3～5厘米。把泡好的中药放在火上，先用大火煮开，然后改用文火慢煮。一般情况是分两次煎煮，第一次煎煮后得到的叫头煎药，将药液倒出，然后再加适量的水，淹没药材2～3厘米左右，进行第二次煎煮。一般一剂中药煎两次就够了，第二次煎煮时间可略短。治疗感冒等的中药煎煮10～15分钟即可，补益类的中药则需煎煮40～60分钟，其余的煎煮20～25分钟即可。煎药时要注意搅拌药料，让药料充分煎煮。为了让药效一致，需要把分次煎好的药混在一起，然后再分开服用。为了节约时间，很多人会一次煎制出几天的药量，服用前再加热药液，但一般不需要煮沸，达到饮用温水的温度即可。另外需要提醒的是，加热中药一般不建议用微波炉。

中药的成分非常复杂，用微波炉加热中药时，产热的过程可能使药材的分子水平遭到破坏，失去一部分功效。

Decocting Chinese medicine refers to a cooking process of putting the prescribed Chinese medicine into a casserole. First, soak the Chinese medicine in cold water for more than 30 minutes. The water should cover the medicine with 3−5 cm high. Put the casserole with soaked Chinese medicine on the fire, boil it with high heat first and then switch to a mild fire. It's usually cooked twice. After first decocting, pour out the liquid, namely "first decocting". Then add the right amount of water and inundate the medicinal material to about 2−3 cm for the second decocting. Generally, it is enough to decoct a dose of Chinese medicine twice. The second time can be slightly short. Herbal remedies for colds and the like can be boiled for 10−15 minutes. Tonic herbs are boiled for 40−60 minutes. 20−25 minutes will do for the others. When decocting medicine, it is necessary to stir the ingredients and let the liquid be fully decocted. In order to have a uniform effect every time you take it, you need to mix both of the decoctions up and then take it separately. To save time, many people make a few days' worth of doses at a time. You don't have to boil the liquid when you reheat it, just reaching the temperature of warm water. What needs to remind additionally is that microwave ovens are not recommended for heating decoction. The ingredients of Chinese medicine are very complex. When heating them in a microwave oven, the process of producing heat may cause the drug to be damaged at the molecular level and some efficacies may be lost.

## 第二节 艾 草
**Mugwort**

艾草与中国人的生活有着密切的关系。艾草是多年生草本或半灌木状植物，有浓烈的香气。民间把它做成枕头，可安眠解乏。也有人把它做成药背心，以防治慢性支气管炎或哮喘及虚寒胃痛等。将艾叶熬成汁，兑水稀释后沐浴，可除身上的小红疙瘩。此外，它还可以驱蚊蝇，灭菌消毒，预防疾病。艾草还用于针灸的"灸"。用艾草泡脚有很多保健功效，特别是在端午节这天乘着露水采到艾草后，药效最好。艾草还是一种食用植物，可作艾叶茶、艾叶汤、艾叶粥、艾草馍、艾草糍粑糕、艾草肉丸等，食用后可增强人体对疾病的抵抗能力。民间有悬艾草的习俗。每到端午节，人们把插艾草和悬菖蒲作为重要活动之一。端午节这天家家都洒扫庭院，把菖蒲、艾条插在门楣，或悬于厅堂来防蚊虫。把菖蒲、艾叶等装入袋中，做成人形或虎形，称为"艾人""艾虎"。或做成花环、佩饰，美丽芬芳，女性朋友们争相佩戴，用来驱瘴。古时候，人们把干枯后的艾草株体泡水进行熏蒸或洗浴，用以消毒止痒。

Mugwort is closely related to Chinese people's life. It is a perennial herb or semi-shrub with a strong aroma. Folk people make it into pillows to sleep well. Medicated vests are also made with it for preventing and curing chronic bronchitis, asthma or stomachache with deficiency and cold pattern. The mugwort leaves are boiled to medicated liquid, which is diluted with water for bathing. The little red bumps on your body can be removed. In addition, it can also drive mosquitoes and flies for sterilization and disinfection. Mugwort is also used in moxibustion. Soaking your feet with it has many health care effects, especially after collecting them with dew on Dragon Boat Festival. Mugwort is also an edible plant that can be made into tea, soup, porridge, buns, glutinous rice cake, meatballs and other recipes for enhancing the human body's resistance to disease. There is a folk custom of hanging mugwort. On Dragon Boat Festival, people hang mugwort and calamus as one of the important activities. Every family sweeps the courtyard, puts calamus and mugwort on the doors or hangs them in the halls to prevent mosquitoes. Bags with calamus and mugwort are made into human or tiger shapes, known as "mugwort figure" and "mugwort tiger" or made into garlands and baldrics with beautiful fragrance which women would like to wear and used to drive miasma. In ancient times, people got fumigated or bathed with the withered stems in water to relieve itching and prevent diseases.

## 第三节 艾 灸
**Moxibustion Regimen**

众所周知，艾灸能够治疗多种疾病，同时也有保健养生功效。但是错误的艾灸操作不仅达不到调理身体的效果，反而可能诱发多种疾病。第一，晚上六点之后艾灸会引起阴阳相冲，影响睡眠质量，甚至会出现失眠多梦。艾灸可以安排在白天。第二，要根据自己的年龄、性别以及承受力来选择不同粗细的艾条，不能一味地追求粗艾条。第三，一些人习惯用水浇灭艾条，认为简单方便，但是这样不安全。正确的方法是把燃烧的艾条直接插在灭火罐里闷5分钟。第四，对于第一次艾灸的人来说，不能艾灸时间太长，应该依据循序渐进的原则，慢慢延长时间。第五，有人认为艾灸越烫越好，但若没有掌握好度的话可能会灼伤或者烫伤皮肤。艾灸有保健养生的功效，主要是因为燃烧的艾能够产生红外能量，这种热能直接渗透到深层的皮下组织。艾条燃烧的时候表面温度高，因此要距离皮肤远一些操作，让局部皮肤稍微感觉到温暖即可。艾条大约燃烧10分钟左右，表面温度降低一些，此时可距离皮肤近一些。

It is well known that moxibustion can assist in the treatment of many diseases as well as health care. But the wrong moxibustion operation cannot achieve the effect of regulating the body, even will cause a variety of diseases. First, moxibustion after 6 o'clock in the evening will cause disharmony of yin and yang, affecting the quality of sleep such as the occurrence of insomnia and dreams. Moxibustion can be scheduled during the day. Second, you have to choose moxa sticks of different sizes according to your age, gender and tolerance. You can't just go for the thick one. Third, some people are used to dousing the mugwort with water, thinking it is simple and convenient, but it is not safe. The correct way is to put the burning strips directly into the fire extinguisher tank and let it cool for 5 minutes. Fourthly, for the first moxibustion, the time should not be too long. You should take a step-by-step approach and wait for your body to get used to it before extending the time. Fifthly, some people think that the hotter moxibustion temperature is, the better. If not properly managed, it can burn your skin. Moxibustion can achieve the effect of health care, mainly because the burning of mugwort can produce infrared energy that directly penetrates into the deep subcutaneous tissue. The burning mugwort has a high surface temperature, so keep it away from the skin at a certain distance. After the moxa stick burns about 10 minutes or so, its surface temperature will decrease a little. At this time you can bring it closer to the skin.

## 第四节 按　摩
**Massage**

自我按摩，对延年益寿是有益处的。当然，前提是要按对地方，用对方法才行。部位一：前胸。建议每天坚持按摩前胸，激活胸腺，可起到防病延年的作用。一般来说，用手掌上下摩擦前胸，摩擦100 ～ 200次即可。部位二：脊柱。脊柱两侧分布的经络，与人体的五脏六腑有着极为密切的关系，经常按摩脊柱附近的穴位，能够疏通经络，促使气血运行、血脉畅通，从而滋养全身的器官。注意了，脊柱可是很重要的地方，不能自己随意按摩，想要按摩的话，要到中医院的推拿科进行按摩。因为非正规的诊所或是养生店，无法确保按摩师的资质，若是对方不够专业的话，按摩之后，也许会造成极大的损伤。部位三：脚底。脚底不仅穴位多，而且在此汇聚的经络也多。脚底分布的末梢神经有成千上万个，它们与大脑、心脏联系十分密切。平常多按摩脚底，可以更好地将远端的血推向心脏和全身，调节体内阴阳平衡，起到防治疾病、健身益寿的功效。按摩脚底方法很多，比如经常弯弯脚趾，踩鹅卵石，穿着袜子在指压板上行走，压脚心等。

It is beneficial to prolong life if one learns to massage himself at ordinary times, of course, as long as you're in the right place and in the right way. Position 1: Forechest. It is recommended to

治疗养生　第八章

massage your chest every day to help activate the thymus gland and prevent disease and prolong life. Generally, rub your front chest up and down with your palms about 100 to 200 times. Position 2: Spine. The meridians distributed on both sides of your spine have a very close relationship with the viscera of the human body. Massaging the nearby acupoints of your spine often can dredge the meridians, leading to the promotion of the flow of qi and blood and unblocked blood vessels, thus nourishing the organs of the whole body. Attention. The spinal column is a very important place. You cannot massage yourself at will. If you want a massage, go to the massage department of the TCM hospital. Informal clinics and health stores do not guarantee the qualification of masseurs. If they are not professional enough, they may cause great damage when you are massaged. Position 3: Soles of feet. The soles of the feet not only have more acupoints, but also more meridians. There are thousands of peripheral nerves in the soles of the feet, which are closely connected with the brain and the heart. Usually massaging your soles of feet can better push the distal blood to the heart and the whole body and regulate the balance of yin and yang in the body. It can prevent and cure diseases, keep fit and prolong life. There are many ways to massage the soles of your feet, such as bending your toes, stepping on pebbles, walking on the fingerboard in your socks and pressing your soles, etc.

## 第五节 刮 痧
### Scraping Regimen

刮痧可以帮助排毒，但是要注意一些小细节才能更好地起到作用。一是刮痧的时候，毛孔处于开放状态，如果被寒风吹到，会直接进入身体，不仅影响刮痧的效果，而且很有可能还会导致疾病。因此，在刮痧后的半小时内，不建议到室外进行活动。另外，等身上的毛孔闭合之后再去洗澡，避免风寒入侵体内，造成感冒等。二是刮痧排毒，要消耗部分体内的津液，刮痧后饮温水一杯，不仅可以补充消耗的部分津液，而且能促进新陈代谢，加速代谢产物的排出。三是刮痧后，要注意饮食清淡，避免过多食用油腻厚重的食物，还要有针对性地调理脏腑。刮痧后皮肤表面会出现红、紫、黑斑或黑疱，称为"出痧"。这些都是背部刮痧后的正常反应，几天以后会自行消失，不用过多担心。四是刮痧不建议空腹，最好在餐后1～2小时后进行。

Scrapping can help discharge toxin, but attention should be paid to some details to get better effects. Firstly, the pores of the skin are in an open state during scrapping. If a cold wind blows into the skin, it will directly enter the body, which will not only affect the scrapping effect, but also possibly cause new diseases. Therefore, you can go outside half an hour later after scrapping. In addition, you should wait for the pores on your body to close before taking a bath so as to avoid the invasion of wind chill into your body, causing common cold and other diseases. Secondly, scrapping makes the pathogenic factors out of the body, which may consume part of the body fluid, so drinking a cup of warm water after scrapping not only can supplement the consumptive part, but also promote metabolism and accelerate the discharge of metabolic products. Thirdly, diet must be light after scrapping. It is advisable to take in balanced nutrition but avoid excessive consumption of heavy food. Besides, red, purple, black spots or black blisters will appear on the skin, which are called "scrapping marks". These are the normal reaction on your back after scrapping, a few days later they will disappear by themselves. Do not worry too much about them. Fourthly, scrapping had better be performed 1 to 2 hours after meals. An empty stomach should be avoided.

# 第六节 拔 罐
## Cupping Regimen

　　在社会迅速发展的今天，人们的生活压力加大，有不少朋友选择中医理疗技术进行调理，拔罐就是其中的一种。拔罐能够解除肌肉或者关节的疼痛，驱除大部分风寒暑湿燥，其余的部分也会随着气血的流通而消散。下面我们就来说说拔罐养生中需要注意的地方。首先，拔罐之后，相应部位会出现很多罐斑，这些罐斑不会立即褪去，要过一段时间才会消失。其次，应控制好拔罐的频率和留罐的时长。两次拔罐间隔时间不能太短，否则会让皮肤受伤而形成重度瘀青而无法褪去，所以适度就好，不要觉得拔罐舒服而经常拔罐。最后，拔火罐之后切记不要立即洗澡，不要着凉，否则无病也可能引起疾病，更有甚者可能加重病情。

　　With the rapid development of society and increase of living pressure, there are many friends who choose Chinese medicine for keeping in good health. Cupping therapy is one of them. It relieves pain in the muscles or joints because most of the pathogenic wind, heat and dampness can be removed. What are not removed dissipates with the flow of qi and blood. Here we talk about some contraindications of the cupping regimen. First of all, after cupping there will be a lot of marks on the back. They will not fade away immediately and it will take a long time for them to disappear.

治疗养生 第八章

89

Secondly, some people do not control the frequency and duration of cupping properly. Do not appeal to cupping too often. People who use cupping often may suffer from skin inflammation and severe bruising that cannot be removed. So just do it in moderation. Finally, do not take a bath at once or catch a cold after cupping. Otherwise, it will cause diseases or even aggravate the disease.

# 第七节 砭 石
## Bian Stones

砭石养生所用的理疗器具包括：砭块、砭板、砭砧、椭圆砭石、砭棒、砭锥、砭镰、砭扣、砭佩和砭珠等。还可以用砭石做成刮痧板。通过擀、压、滚、擦、刺、划、叩、刮、扭、旋、振、拔、温、凉等手法，进行局部理疗。施砭术时，根据个人的情况选择适当大小的砭具刺激穴位，即点穴位，不是针刺而是采用砭具刺激穴位中点，不必刺穿皮肤。另一种，可在皮肤上施熨法，熨似灸，但又不灼伤皮肤。还有摩法，摩即按法，摩圆周形或反复运作，但不振动骨骼深部。以上均以手操作砭具活动为要点，手到而病除。此外，还可以戴砭石吊坠、手链、项链、腰带等，利用砭石所发出的远红外和超声波脉冲，促进局部的血液循环，有病治病，无病强身。家中也可以摆放砭石磬、砭石编钟、砭石琴等，造型古雅高贵，既精致，又能敲击使之发出优美动听的声音及超声波脉冲，一人击磬，全家听，能使家庭和睦、快乐、健康。

In recent years, more and more people have resorted to bian stones for health care. Here are various forms of bian stones: rock, board, anvil, elliptical stone, stick, awl, sickle, button, pendant, bead, etc. You can also use bian stones to make scraping boards. By rolling, pressing, push-rolling, rubbing, stabbing, scratching, tapping, scraping, twisting, rotating, vibrating, drawing, warming, cooling, etc., local physiotherapy can be performed. In the process of manipulation, the appropriate size of a tool is selected according to the individual's situation to stimulate the acupoints, that is, to press the points. Instead of needling, the stimulation should focus on the midpoint without penetrating the skin. Another method applied to the skin is ironing like moxibustion, but it does not burn the skin. And still, rubbing, meaning pressing, is operated in a circular or back-and-forth way, but the vibration should not be performed deep into the bone. All of the above activities focus on manual operations to get rid of disease. In addition, one can wear pendants, bracelets, necklaces and belts that are made of this material. The infrared and ultrasonic pulses sent out by bian stones are used to promote local blood circulation so as to cure diseases and strengthen health. You can also put a chime and a harp made of this kind of stone at home. They are elegant in shape and can be struck to send out beautiful and pleasant sounds and ultrasonic pulse. Striking a stone chime and listening to its rhythm can bring a family with harmony, happiness and health.

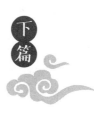

下篇

感悟篇

PART III
GNOSIS

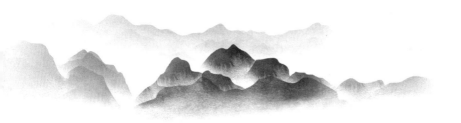

# 考古文物
# Medical Relics

## 第一节　中国最早瘟疫的记载
### The Earliest Recorded Pestilence in China

人类与瘟疫斗争的历史源远流长，早在三千多年前的殷墟甲骨文中，就有了关于瘟疫的记载。有一段商王得了疑似瘟疫的甲骨卜辞，记录在一个牛肩胛骨上，意思是：疫情突发，众人为了除疠疫举行了一系列祭祀先人的活动。这可以说是世界上最早的关于瘟疫的文字记载了。这里的"疫"是"民皆病"的意思，说明在殷商时期，我国已出现过足以致命的传染病，而且它们都得到了上层的充分重视。那么，殷人得了瘟疫如何治疗呢？一是占卜。二是祭祀。三是针刺、灸疗、隔离等。甲骨文中记录的"有疾病者，分而治之"就是在讲隔离措施，说明当时人们对瘟疫相当恐惧，但并非无所作为，他们已经有了隔离防控疫情的应对手段。四是熏燎防疫。进行熏燎室屋门道与野外的祭祀活动。用草熏燎除蛊驱虫来防疫的方法，流传到后世一直不衰。这说明在殷商时期，人们已经能利用某些植物药材来驱除疫疾了。甲骨文所记载的殷商统治者理性实施的疫情防控应对措施，对现代仍有借鉴意义。

The human struggle against epidemics has a long history. As early as 3,000 years ago, there were records of epidemics in the inscriptions on bones or tortoise shells in the Ruins of Yin in China. Some inscriptions on an oracle bone related to the King of the Shang Dynasty who was suspected to be plague-infected were recorded on the shoulder blades of a bull, literally meaning: on the outbreak of the epidemic, the court hosted a series of sacrifices to its ancestors to avoid the pest. This is the earliest written record of the plague in the world. The word "epidemic" here means "all the people are suffering from diseases", which indicates that in the Yin and Shang Dynasties, deadly infectious diseases had appeared in their country and they all got the full attention of the upper class. So how should the Yin people be treated for epidemics? There were such methods as divination, sacrifice, acupuncture and moxibustion therapy, isolation and other active therapies. The oracle-bone inscriptions about "separate and treat those who are sick" refer to the measure of isolation which was a sign that people were fearful of the epidemic, but not inactive. They had the measures in place to isolate the sick and stop rumors that might cause the panic. Another method is fumigation for epidemic prevention. Fume the rooms and doorway and carry on the sacrificial activity in the field. The method of controlling evils by means of grass fumigation or repelling insects has been passed down to later generations. This shows that in the Shang Dynasty, people could have already used some plants as medicine to get rid of epidemic diseases. The measures rationally implemented by the Yin and Shang rulers recorded on the oracle bones are of great significance for modern times.

## 第二节 绵阳双包山汉针灸人模型
### The Han Acupuncture Figure at Shuangbao Mountain, Mianyang

　　1993年，四川绵阳出土了一具高28.1厘米的木质涂漆的针灸人模型，此模型比北宋王惟一的铜人早1000多年。模型出土时身裹数层红色纺织物，木胎，黑漆，裸体直立，手臂伸直，掌心向前，左手和右脚略残，造型写实。值得注意的是，它的体表纵向分布着数条红色线条。人体正面从头顶，经胸腹，到脚有两条主线；背面则有三根线条，两根从头顶经背部到脚，另外一根从头顶向下至臀缝；两腋经大腿外侧到外踝各垂直分布一线条；两臂各有五根线条，从指尖，经手臂到颈部，与头部线条连接，形成网络；头部和手臂线条最为复杂，头部正面纵线五根，与头部侧面耳前纵线条相连，再与两外眼角横出的各三根线条形成交织复杂的网络。这些遍布于全身的经脉循行路径，在黑漆的烘托下，格外清晰分明，使人容易辨识。这是迄今为止，不仅在中国，也是在世界上所发现的最古老的标有经脉流注的木质人体模型。它为研究我国人体经脉的起源、经脉学理论的初步形成和发展，提供了珍贵的实物资料。

　　In 1993, a wooden and painted acupuncture figure of 28.1cm tall was unearthed in Mianyang, Sichuan Province. This model is more than 1000 years earlier than the Bronze Figure of Wang Weiyi in the Northern Song Dynasty. When unearthed, it was covered with layers of red fabric and painted black, standing upright and naked. Its right arm is straight with its palm forward. His left hand and right foot are slightly damaged. The overall shape is realistic. In particular, it has several red lines on its body surface. There are two main lines on its front from the top of the head through the chest and abdomen to the feet. It has three lines on the back with two running from the top of the head down to the feet and the other one running from the top of the head down to the hips. From the two armpits through the lateral thighs to the lateral ankles is vertically distributed a line respectively. There are five lines on each arm, running from the fingertip, through the arm to the neck and connected to the line of the head to form a network. The lines on the head and arms are the most complex. There are five longitudinal lines on the front of the head, which are connected with the longitudinal lines in front of the ear on the side of the head, and then form an interwoven and complex network with the three lines from each outer canthus. These meridians all over the body beneath the black paint of skin are very clear and easy to recognize. This is by far the oldest wooden mannequin marked with the meridians found not only in China but also in the world. It provides the valuable physical material for the study of the origin of human body meridians and the preliminary formation and development of the meridian theory.

## 第三节　跨湖桥新石器时代茎枝类草药遗存
## The Stems and Branches of Herbs Remains at the Neolithic Age

　　跨湖桥文化遗址是浙江省境内最早的新石器时代文化遗址。这一发现，把浙江的文明史提前到了8000年前的新石器时代早期，是浙江悠久的历史和深厚的文化积淀的重要证据。2001年，考古工作者对跨湖桥遗址进行了发掘，出土了一大批陶、石、骨、木器，其中有一件稍有残缺的绳纹小陶釜，口径11.3厘米、高8.8厘米，外底有烟火熏焦痕，器内盛有一捆植物茎枝，长度约5～8厘米，单根直径在0.3～0.8厘米之间，共20余根，纹理清晰，出土时头尾整齐地摆在釜底。从这些现象观察，可以判断是因陶釜烧裂而丢弃的。植物标本被送到浙江省药品检验所中药室检测，鉴定为茎枝类草药。传说商初重臣尹伊发明了草药煎剂，这次出土的文物对研究我国中草药的起源，尤其是煎药的起源具有重要的价值。在处于新石器时代的浙江萧山跨湖桥遗址中，考古学家发现了盛有煎煮过草药的小陶釜，说明史前期人们已认识到自然中植物的药用价值。

　　The cultural relics site of the Bridge across the Lake is the earliest neolithic cultural site in Zhejiang Province. The discovery pushed Zhejiang's civilization back 8,000 years to the early Neolithic period thus an important evidence of the province's long history and deep cultural accumulation. In 2001, the archaeologists excavated a large number of potteries, stones, bones and wooden objects, including a small jomon pot with a slight defect, 11.3 cm in diameter and 8.8 cm in height. There are scorch marks on its outer bottom and a bundle of plant branches inside. They are about 5-8 cm long and the diameter of a single one is generally between 0.3-0.8 cm. There are more than 20 branches in total with clear texture. When unearthed, they were neatly placed in the bottom of the kettle. From the observation of these remains, it can be concluded that they are decoctions discarded due to the cracking of the pottery kettle. The specimen was sent to the TCM Laboratory of Zhejiang Provincial Institute for Drug Control and identified as the herbal stems. It is said that Yi Yin, a high-ranking official of the early Shang Dynasty, invented the decocted herbal medicine. These herbs unearthed indicate that they are of great value to the study of the origin of Chinese herbal medicine, especially the origin of decoctions. On the Neolithic site of the Bridge across the Lake in Xiaoshan, Zhejiang, the archaeologists discovered a small pottery kettle containing decocted herbs, indicating that ancient people had long recognized the medicinal value of plants in nature.

## 第四节　老官山汉墓医学文物
### Medical Relics of Laoguan Mountain Han Tombs

### 老官山汉经穴髹漆人像

Painted Meridian Figure of the Han Dynasty in Laoguan Mountain

老官山汉墓出土的经穴髹漆人像高约14厘米，其五官肢体刻画得准确，人像身体上清晰可见用白色或红色描绘的经络线条和穴点，共有22条红线、29条白线，用以标识经脉、任脉和带脉。与《灵枢·经脉》记载的十二经脉分布相似，漆木人共有117个穴位，还刻有"心""肺""肾"等小字，有文字标记的是针刺治疗的重要部位，专家推断是用来提示解剖的部位或提醒医师针治这些部位时应格外小心。经穴髹漆人像是迄今为止我国发现的最早、最完整的经穴人体医学模型。对解开中华医学经络理论的起源具有重要意义，这也证明在西汉早期中医针灸学已经形成了较完整的理论体系。1993年，在绵阳出土的经络漆人，是世界上发现最早的标有经脉流注的木质人体模型，其年代比老官山汉墓的经穴髹漆人像略早，但绵阳的经络漆人只有经脉而没有穴位，而老官山汉墓出土的人像，既有经脉标注，又有穴位的标注。据史料记载，北宋有针灸铜人作为教具，但并没有实物留存于世，所以此次发现的早于北宋1000年的西汉时期人像模型就更显珍贵了。

The Painted Meridian Figure, unearthed from the Han Tombs in Laoguan Mountain, is about 14cm tall with its facial features and limbs accurately delineated. The meridians and acupoints depicted in white or red can be clearly seen on the figure. There are 22 red lines and 29 white lines to identify the meridians. Ren and Dai meridians are similar to those recorded in *Lingshu · Meridians*. There are 117 points in total with some small characters such as "heart", "lung" and "kidney" engraved on them. The important parts are marked with words for acupuncture presumably to indicate the anatomical part or to remind the manipulator of needling these parts carefully. The Painted Meridian Figure is the earliest and most complete medical model, which is of great significance to untangle the origin of the acupuncture theory of Chinese medicine and also proves that acupuncture in the early Western Han Dynasty has formed a relatively complete theoretical system. The Meridian Figure unearthed in Mianyang in 1993, is the earliest wooden figure marked with the meridians in the world. It is a little earlier than the Painted Meridian Figure in Laoguan Mountain. The Mianyang Figure only has meridians and no acupoints, but the figure unearthed in Laoguan Mountain marks the meridians and acupoints. According to historical records, there were bronze figures with acupuncture as the teaching tools in the Northern Song Dynasty, but no physical objects remained in the world, so it is extremely precious to have such a model in the Western Han Dynasty 1,000 years before the Northern Song Dynasty.

## 老官山汉医简

The Medical Bamboo Slips of the Han Dynasty in Laoguan Mountain

成都老官山汉墓出土的西汉时期的医简是一项重要发现，被考古专家认为极有可能是扁鹊学派的经典书籍。九部医书涉及了中医学的多门学科，既有中医理论，又有症候的治疗、针灸、脉诊等，包括内科、外科、妇科、皮肤科、五官科、伤科等，甚至还有医治马匹的兽医书。此前，马王堆汉墓、张家山汉墓也曾出土过医学文献，但成都老官山出土的医简，是数量最大、最集中、与医学关系最密切。马王堆出土的医书的内容有很多原始、巫术的成分，医方也以单方为主，经验的成分比较大。成都老官山出土的医简比马王堆出土的医书更加成熟，除了经方外，还有复方，说明中医已经走向发展的轨道，其在医学史上的价值，远远高于马王堆医书。从药方组成来看，有了君臣佐使的基本结构以及中医辨证施治的原理，是中医药开始成熟的标志。专家们认为，老官山汉墓出土的医简中，没有巫术的描述，这证明了在西汉早中期医巫已经分家。

The Han Tombs in Laoguan Mountain, Chengdu, were discovered in 2013, in which the Western Han medical bamboo slips unearthed were an important discovery. They are considered by the archaeologists to be the classic books of Bian Que School. The unearthed nine medical books cover many disciplines of traditional Chinese medicine, including TCM theory, treatment of symptoms, acupuncture, pulse diagnosis, etc., namely internal medicine, surgery, gynecology, dermatology, ENT, orthopedics and traumatology, etc., as well as veterinary books for treating horses. Previously, medical documents were unearthed from the Han Tombs in Mawangdui and Zhangjiashan, but the medical bamboo slips in Laoguan Mountain in Chengdu have the largest quantity with the most concentrated and closely related to medicine in the history of TCM. Mawangdui's medical books contain a lot of primitive and sorcery elements and their recorded prescriptions are mainly single-herb ones. The prescriptions of Chengdu Laoguan Mountain in the medical bamboo slips are more mature than those of Mawangdui's medical books. Besides the classic prescriptions, there are also compound prescriptions of multiple herbs, indicating that TCM then had been on the track of independent development. The value of this batch of medical bamboo slips in the history of medicine is much higher than that of Mawangdui's medical books. In terms of the compositions of these prescriptions, they reflect the functional roles of monarch, minister, assistant and guide of medications as well as the therapeutic principles of dialectical therapy in Chinese medicine, which is a good illustration of the beginning of TCM maturity. Experts believe that the absence of any description of witchcraft in the medical bamboo slips unearthed from the Han Tombs in Laoguan Mountain proves that "medicine" and "witchcraft" were separated in the early and mid-Western Han Dynasty.

考古文物 第九章

105

## 第五节　灸艾图
### *The Painting of Moxibustion*

宋代李唐笔下的《灸艾图》描绘了走方郎中为贫苦百姓治病的情形。村舍、小桥、柳树、土坡，构成了典型的乡村田园风景；底层的劳动人民，衣衫散乱不整，到处是补丁，面容清瘦，连走方郎中也是衣衫褴褛，身材可能是因常年劳作而有些驼背。树荫下，病人正经受着痛苦，只见他袒露着上身，双臂被一老农妇和一个少年紧紧地抓着，他双眼圆瞪、张着嘴，声嘶力竭地喊着，一条伸出的腿也被人死死踩住，这时的他，只能听凭背上的疮伤被艾火熏灼。他那绷紧的肌肉、散乱的衣服、紧皱的眉头，说明这痛苦已达到了极点。老农妇手拽脚踩地协助着医生，脸上显露着对病人深情的怜悯和愁苦神色。两个少年对病人的叫喊和医生的"狠手"难以忍受，一个把脸藏到老妇背后，一个眯起一只眼，像是既不敢看又关心治疗过程。医生手中操作着，嘴里似乎说些安慰的话。医生身后，一个小学徒手里正捧着一个大帖膏药，对它呵着气，准备灸艾一完便贴到病人的疮口上去。

*The Painting of Moxibustion*, created by Li Tang in the Song Dynasty, depicts how a practitioner treated a poor patient. In the picture, cottages, small bridges, willows and slopes constituted a typical rural idyllic scenery. The labouring patient was ragged and patched with a thin face and even the doctor was disheveled and patched with his figure crooked due to years of work. Under the shade of a tree, the patient was undergoing a painful ordeal. He was stripped to his waist with his arms tightly held by an old woman and a young boy. His eyes were wide and his mouth was open, screaming at the top of his lungs. One of his outstretched legs was crushed. At this time, he could only allow the sore on his back by moxibustion fire burning. His taut muscles, dishevelled clothes and frowning brows showed that his pain had reached its climax. The old woman assisted the practitioner and her face was full of deep pity and distress for the sick man. The patient's screams and the doctor's "cruelty" were too much for the boys to bear. One hid his face behind the old woman while the other squinted one eye as if he neither dared to look nor cared about the treatment. As he worked, the doctor seemed to say something reassuring. Behind the practitioner, a little apprentice was holding a large plaster in his bare hands, breathing on it and preparing to put it on the patient's wound as soon as the moxibustion was finished.

考古文物 第九章

## 第六节　明代民间传世针灸铜人
## The Bronze Figure Marked with Acupoints of the Ming Dynasty

　　明代民间传世针灸铜人是一个古代童子的形象，高86.5厘米，全身穴位数百个。每个穴位对应一个针孔，旁边刻有该穴位的名称。铜人呈半跪姿势，左手上举，右手下垂。据推测，相比其他铜人的直立形象，采取这种姿势的原因在于腿部和足部的穴位众多，经络循行路线复杂，如果和其他铜人一样采取站立姿势，则难以看清一些被遮挡部位的腧穴和经络，不便于针灸教学。这件铜像还被设计成旋转样式，更利于教学观察。值得注意的是，该铜人左手上举的奇特的手掌姿势，其实是显示了中医针灸中的"中指同身寸"的手法。所谓"中指同身寸"手法，是中医针灸中的一种取穴方法，是以患者的中指长度或宽度折作若干等分以量取穴位。这个针灸铜人在设计时，还十分注重骨性标志，其胸背肋骨、肩胛骨相当明显。骨性标志是腧穴定位的重要标记，在骨节的突起或凹陷处往往分布有重要的腧穴。骨性标志如此突出的针灸铜人除这件外，仅有韩国收藏的针灸铜人和日本东京国立博物馆收藏的江户时期的铜人。

　　The bronze figure marked with the acupoints handed down from the Ming Dynasty, is an image of an ancient boy with 86.5

centimeters tall and hundreds of acupoints all over his body. Each acupoint has a pinhole and a name inscribed beside it. The bronze figure keeps in a semi-kneeling position with his left hand raised and his right hand hanging. It is speculated that compared with other bronze figures, the reason for this posture is that there are many acupoints in the legs and feet and the complicated circulation of the meridians. If it takes a standing posture like other bronze figures, it is difficult for people to see some occluded parts of the acupoints and meridians, which is not conducive to acupuncture teaching. The statue is also designed to rotate so that it can be observed more easily by learners. It is worth noting that the peculiar gesture of the palm held on the bronze figure's left hand actually shows the "cun as a measurement with one's upper part of the middle finger" technique in acupuncture. The so-called "cun as a measurement with one's upper part of the middle finger" technique is a method, in which the length of the patient's middle finger is folded into several equal parts to locate the acupoints. In the design of the bronze figure, attention is paid to its bone features of quite obvious chest, back ribs and shoulder blades. The bone feature is very important for the location of acupoints because there are often important acupoints in the protrusions or depressions of the joints. Besides this one, the only bronze figure in Korea and bronze figure of the Edo period in the National Museum of Tokyo, Japan have such prominent bony features.

# 第七节　敦煌医学宝库
## The Treasure House of Dunhuang Medicine

### 敦煌藏经洞中医药文献宝库
Dunhuang Cave as the Treasure House of TCM Literature

在敦煌藏经洞中，关于医学的卷子有100种以上，涉及医理类、诊法类、本草类、针灸类等各个方面。其中，《灸经图》是我国现存较早的灸法专著。因其与传世医书内容不同且历代医籍未见收载，也一直成为各医家研究的重点。专家们认为，《灸经图》中所倡导的治疗疑难重病的重灸思想对后世医学发展影响深远，值得今人进一步挖掘整理和推广应用。在敦煌文献中，保存有我国第一部官颁药典——唐《新修本草》残卷。这是唐高宗年间，唐朝政府组织人员编写的一部医药学大典，图文并茂，共记载药物800多种，是此前一千多年我国药物学知识的集大成之作，在宋代失传，后来有人在日本发现该书的部分残本。同样，在宋代后失传的唐代食疗著作《食疗本草》，也神奇地出现在敦煌遗书中。这部引人注目的医药学残卷共收录药物200多种，以动植物营养和药用医疗价值为特色。尽管敦煌出土的《食疗本草》仅存药物26种，约为原书的十分之一，却有着极高的价值，为了解唐代人对食疗的认识提供了难得的资料。

In Dunhuang Sutra Caves, there were over 100 kinds of medical records, covering medical theories, diagnostic methods, herbal medicine, acupuncture and moxibustion, etc. *The Meridians With Moxibustion* was one of the earliest monographs of moxibustion in China. Because its different contents from the medical books handed down in previous dynasties have not been collected, it has always been the focus of medical researchers. Experts believe that the idea of severe moxibustion for the treatment of difficult diseases advocated in *The Meridians With Moxibustion* had a profound influence on the medical development of later generations and it is worth further exploring, organizing and popularizing. In Dunhuang documents, there are the residual volumes of the preserved China's first official pharmacopoeia — "*New Revised Materia Medica*" of the Tang Dynasty, which was a pharmacology canon compiled by the government in the reign of the Emperor Gaozong of the Tang Dynasty. It records more than 800 kinds of medicines with pictures and illustrations. It had been a collective masterpiece of Chinese pharmacology for more than 1,000 years before that. Then, it was lost in the Song Dynasty with parts of the book later found in Japan. Similarly, *Dietotherapy of Materia Medica* of the Tang Dynasty got lost after the Song Dynasty, which magically appeared in the Dunhuang relics. More than 200 medicines are included in this remarkable medical collection, which features on the nutritional and medicinal value of plants and animals. Although there are only 26 kinds of medicinal herbs in the manuscript unearthed in Dunhuang, which is about one tenth of the original book, it is of great value and provides rare materials for understanding the Tang people on food therapy.

考古文物

第九章

111

## 敦煌医学

Dunhuang Medicine

敦煌医学是一门关于整理和研究敦煌藏经洞遗书、敦煌壁画以及其他敦煌文物的学科。目前，敦煌文献除国家图书馆藏有一万余卷外，其余都被当时英、法、俄、日等国的探险者所夺，分别收藏于英国国家图书馆、法国国立图书馆以及德国、俄国、日本、美国、印度等地。据研究，现存于国内外的敦煌医学卷子大约有100种以上，其内容涉及医经、五脏、诊法、伤寒、医方、本草、针灸、养生等方面。这些医学文献的年代多撰成于六朝及以前，也有部分是隋唐时期的医学文献。这些文献中包括许多长期失传的医药古籍，以及一些流传至今的古籍的最早传抄本。它们最能反映早期医学文献的原貌，因而对研究中国医药发展史，澄清医药文献的部分疑难问题，以及对校勘、补缺和探求宋以后木刻本的源流，都具有非常重要的价值。20世纪有关敦煌医学文献的研究日益增多并不断深化。随着世界敦煌学的发展和科学技术的进步，世界各国陆续对敦煌出土文献进行了影印出版，大大促进了敦煌文献的研究进展。

Dunhuang medicine is a discipline concerned with the collation and study of the remains of Dunhuang scripture caves, Dunhuang frescoes and other Dunhuang cultural relics. At present, the Dunhuang documents are collected in the National Library of England, the National Library of France, Germany, Russia, the United States, India and other countries, except for the National Library of China which contains more than 10,000 volumes. According to research, there are over 100 kinds of Dunhuang medical records existing at home and abroad, which cover such aspects as medical classics, five zang-organs, diagnostic methods, typhoid fever, medical prescriptions, herbal medicine, acupuncture and moxibustion, health preservation, etc. Most of these medical documents were written in the Six Dynasties and before and some of them were from the Sui and Tang dynasties. These documents include many long-lost ancient medical books as well as some of the earliest handwritten copies of ancient books that have survived to this day. They can best reflect the original appearance of early medical literature, so they are of great value in studying the development history of Chinese medicine, clarifying some difficult problems in medical literature, and correcting, filling in and exploring the origin and development of woodcut books after the Song Dynasty. In the 20th century, the research on Dunhuang medical literature is increasing and deepening. With the development of Dunhuang studies in the world and the progress of scientific technology, some countries in the world have successively photocopied and published Dunhuang unearthed documents, thus promoting the study of Dunhuang documents.

考古文物 第九章

## 敦煌藏经洞医书——美容方

The Library Cave in Dunhuang － The Beauty Prescription

在敦煌藏经洞发现的唐代民间传抄本医书中，录有烧炼益母草灰以消除脸上黑斑、粉刺、癣疮等的方子。草木灰呈碱性，能够去除油污，因此一直是人们洗涤衣物、清洁身体的重要物品之一。益母草灰是一种草木灰碱。益母草灰美容的方法早在唐代就被广为流传，而且益母草灰美容并不是宫廷贵妇们独享的专利，而是一项生活常识。在南宋末年的生活百科全书《事林广记》中，益母草灰更是发展为一种可配有多种中草药成分的复合型制品。人们用茯苓、天门冬、香附子、甘草、杏仁、皂角、大豆等与益母草搭配，用于洗面、祛瘢疮。还将益母草灰制成碱皂。固体皂在唐代初见雏形，不过，是宋人发明了用肥皂角与中药调和而成的固体清洁皂，从此各种皂角制成的固体皂成为中国人的主要美容清洁用品。明代的美容专书《香奁润色》中，便出现了一款由益母草和肥皂组成的"治美人面上粉刺方"。

In the medical books popular among the people in the Tang Dynasty, which were found in the Dunhuang Sutra Cave, there were prescriptions for burning motherwort ashes to eliminate black spots, acne, tinea and other problems on the face.

In traditional culture, plant ash has been one of the most

important items for people to wash clothes and clean their bodies because it contains alkalinity and can remove oil stains. Motherwort ash is a kind of grass ash alkali which was used for beauty to be spread widely as early as the Tang Dynasty. It was not the exclusive preserve of court ladies, but a common sense of life for the majority of ordinary women to be familiar with. In the encyclopedia of life *"Shi Lin Guang Ji"* in the late Southern Song Dynasty, motherwort ash developed into a compound product with various Chinese herbal ingredients. Poria, lucid asparagus, nutgrass galingale rhizome, licorice root, almond, saponin and soybean were used to mix motherwort for cleansing face and removing blemishes. Moreover, motherwort ash was also made into alkali soap. Solid soaps first appeared in the Tang Dynasty, but it was people of the Song Dynasty who invented the solid cleaning soap made of Chinese honey locust and Chinese medicine. Since then, solid soaps made of various Chinese honey locusts have become the main beauty and cleaning products for the Chinese people. Later, in the beauty book *"Xianglian Runse"* of the Ming Dynasty, there was a "prescription for beauty acne" made of motherwort and soap.

## 第八节　满城汉医学文物
## The Medical Relics in the Mancheng Han Tombs

　　满城出土的医疗器具在汉代考古史上十分罕见。其中有金针4枚、银针5枚，是用来针刺经络的，是现存最早的金银针。金针包括1枚金锋针、2枚金毫针和1枚金鍉针。"医工盆"口径27.6厘米、高8.3厘米，以铜制成，盆的口沿刻有"医工"字样。"医工"即医者，汉代诸侯王国主管医务的官吏称为"医工长"。盆的口部和底部各有一处修补，用铜钉铆合。此盆是中山王刘胜内府所用，是年代最早而自铭为医用的器具，在中国医学史上有重要价值。灌药器和漏斗据推测是配套使用的医疗用具。灌药器是带长嘴的小壶，壶身呈扁圆形，有盖，盖与壶身由能转动的钮相连。此壶用于为危重昏迷不能自行进食的病人灌喂药食。漏斗则用于向灌药器中注入汤药。另外，还有铜手术刀等文物，为中国医学史的研究增添了宝贵的实物资料。铜捣药杵、铜药匙，说明汉代医疗对药物的剂型、剂量已经有了严格的要求。水晶砭石用来刺激体表部位，或用于放血排脓。这些医学文物是中医学发展的重要物证。

The medical relics unearthed in Mancheng are very rare in archaeology. Four gold needles and five silver needles are used to puncture the meridians. They are the earliest gold and silver needles seen so far. The gold needles include one gold three-edged needle, two gold filiform needles and one gold thick needle. The "medical basin" is 27.6 cm in diameter and 8.3 cm tall. It is made of copper and the word "medical worker" meaning the physician is engraved along the edge of the basin. The officials in charge of medical treatment in the Han Dynasty were called "the chief medical worker". Due to the long-term use, the mouth and bottom of the basin have repairs riveted with copper. This basin, used by Liu Sheng, the king of Zhongshan, is the earliest utensil with its name as a medical appliance. It is of great value in the history of Chinese medicine. The drencher and funnel are presumed to be the complementary medical appliances. The drencher is a small pot with a long spowt. Its body is flat and round with a cover, which is connected with the body by a knob that can be turned. This pot was used to administer medicine to the critically ill and unconscious patients who couldn't feed themselves. The funnel was used to pour the medicinal liquid into the drencher. In addition, the copper scalpel and other cultural relics have added valuable physical materials to the study of Chinese medical history. The copper pestle and spoon show that there were strict requirements on the drug dosage in treatment in the Han Dynasty. The crystal bian stone was used to stimulate the surface of the body or to bleed and discharge pus. These medical relics are not eye-catching, but they are important witnesses of the development of Chinese medicine.

# 第九节　武威汉代医简
## The Medical Bamboo and Wooden Slips in the Wuwei Han Tombs

　　东汉医学简牍，共有92片，其中竹简78片，木牍14片。简牍详细地记载了病名、症状、药物、剂量、制药方法、服药时间以及不同的用药方式，还记述了一些穴位、针刺禁忌等，内容极为丰富，是迄今为止我们所能见到的汉简中有关医药方面的最完整的原始资料。简文中还记载着人从1岁到100岁的各个不同年龄阶段，针刺禁忌的器官、部位。这批医学简牍共记录了比较完整的医方30余个，几乎全是复方，一个方剂少则1～2味药，多则15～16味药，说明复方在当时的临床治疗中普遍应用。涉的药物近百种，绝大多数都产自西北地区。尤其值得一提的是，其中有1枚木牍不仅写有药物的名称、剂量，还列出了当时药物的价格，可以帮助我们了解东汉时期的中药材贸易的信息。从辨证论治的水平上分析，武威汉代医简处在初期阶段。武威汉代医简是我国最早的医药学文献之一，对研究甘肃河西地区汉代经济、文化、民情等方面的情况都具有深远的意义。

　　There are a total of 92 medical bamboo and wooden slips of the Eastern Han Dynasty, including 78 bamboo slips and 14 wooden strips. They record in detail the disease names, the symptoms, the drugs, the dosages, the methods of making drugs, the time and different ways of taking drugs. They also describe some acupuncture points, taboos of acupuncture and so on, which are very rich in content. They are the most complete original data about medicine in the bamboo and wooden slips of the Han Dynasty that we have seen so far. The notes also say that at different ages from one to 100, attention should be paid to contraindicated organ areas with acupuncture. This batch of slips records more than 30 relatively complete medical prescriptions, almost all of which are compound, with as a few as 1−2 herbs in one prescription and as many as 15−16 ones, indicating that compound prescriptions had become a common method of clinical treatment at that time. The vast majority of the nearly 100 drugs involved were produced in the Northwest of China. It is worth mentioning that one of the wooden slips not only contains the name and dose of the medicine, but also lists its price at that time, which can help us understand the information of the trade of Chinese medicinal materials in the Eastern Han Dynasty. Wuwei slips show an early-stage development of treatment based on syndrome differentiation in Chinese medicine. The medical bamboo and wooden slips in the Wuwei Han tombs are one of the earliest medical documents in China, which is of great significance to the study of economy, culture and people's living conditions in Hexi area of Gansu Province.

## 第十节　长沙马王堆医学文物
## Medical Relics of the Mawangdui Han Tombs in Changsha

### 长沙马王堆汉《导引图》

*The Picture of Physical and Breathing Exercises* of the
Mawangdui Han Tombs in Changsha

　　马王堆出土的《导引图》是现存最早的道家保健运动的彩色帛画，是西汉早期的作品。图上描绘了44个不同年龄、性别的人物在做不同的运动，人物各个栩栩如生，旁边还注有动作的名称，以及动物形象或器械运动等名称。"导引"是呼吸运动和躯体运动相结合的一种医疗体育方法。早在原始时代，先民们为了表示欢乐、祝福和庆功，往往学着动物的跳跃姿势和飞翔姿势进行舞蹈，后来逐步发展成为锻炼身体的保健方法。《导引图》年代早，内容非常丰富，是最早的图形资料，为导引研究提供了可贵的线索。《导引图》中除极个别的蹲、跪式外，其余全部为立式运动。在《导引图》中还发现使用棍仗的运动，人物双手持杖，作屈身转体的运动。还有折腰式转体运动，人物脚下有一球状物，考古专家推测是用于运动的器械。导引图足以说明中国是世界上较早应用导引的国家。

*The Picture of Physical and Breathing Exercises*, unearthed in the Mawangdui Han Tombs, is the earliest extant painting on silk about Taoist health care movement and an early work of the Western Han Dynasty. The picture depicts 44 people of different ages and genders doing different sports, with lifelike characters and names of movements, including those expressed in animal images or apparatus sports. The so-called "daoyin" is a kind of fitness method combining breathing and body movement. As early as in primitive times, the ancestors often imitated the jumping posture and flying postures of animals for dancing in order to show their joy, blessing and celebration. Later, it gradually developed into a medical method to exercise the body. The *Picture of Physical and Breathing Exercises* is not only antique, but also rich in content. It makes the earliest graphic data of various daoyin and fitness exercises scattered in ancient literature and provides valuable clues to the research of daoyin. In the picture, all the exercises are standing movements except the very few squat and kneeling ones. One figure dose chest dilation and raises his hands back, presumably as a cardiorespiratory workout. A movement with a stick is also found in the picture, in which the figure holds a stick in both hands and bends and turns. There is also the bending movement. The figure has a ball at the foot, which the experts infers that it is an apparatus for exercise. The *Picture of Physical and Breathing Exercises* is sufficient to show that China is one of the early countries applying daoyin in the world.

## 长沙马王堆汉《五十二病方》

*The Fifty-two Prescriptions* from the Mawangdui Han Tombs in Changsha

经考证，《五十二病方》成书比《黄帝内经》（成书于春秋战国时代）可能还要早。全书一万余字，分52个主题，每个主题治疗一类疾病，少则一、二方，多则二十余方。其中涉及医方283个，药物247种，将近半数是东汉时期《神农本草经》中未记载的。书中提到的病名有103个，所治疗的疾病范围包括内、外、妇、儿、五官各科，是我国现存最早的方剂。内科病在全书中所占篇幅不大，这也从一定程度上反映了当时治疗内科病的水平。全书以外科病所占篇幅为最大，也最为突出。《五十二病方》在论述痔疮的治疗时，除了运用各种药物疗法外，还记载了精彩的手术疗法。其他所载的治法多种多样，除了以内服汤药为主之外，还有大量的外治法，如敷贴法、烟熏或蒸气熏法、熨法、砭法、灸法、按摩疗法、角法（火罐疗法）等。治疗手段的多样化，也是当时医疗水平提高的标志之一。《五十二病方》的发现，补充了《黄帝内经》以前的医学内容，是非常珍贵的医学遗产。

*The Fifty-two Prescriptions*, verified by historical data, may be earlier than the *Yellow Emperor's Inner Canon* (written in the Spring and Autumn Period and Warring States Period), with more than 10,000 characters. The book is divided into 52 themes, each of which treats a kind of disease, ranging from one or two to more than 20 prescriptions. It involves a total of 283 prescriptions and 247 medicines, nearly half of which were not recorded in the Shennong's Classic of Materia Medica in the Eastern Han Dynasty. There are 103 diseases mentioned in the book including diseases of internal medicine, surgery, gynecology, pediatrics and facial organs. This is the earliest record of prescriptions that can be seen in our country now. The treatment of internal diseases occupies a small proportion in the book which reflects the level of treatment of internal diseases at that time. The proportion of surgical diseases in the book is the largest and the most prominent. When discussing the treatment of hemorrhoids, "*Fifty-two Prescriptions*" also recorded excellent surgical therapy in addition to the use of a variety of drug therapies. Other treatments are various e.g. a large number of external treatments such as paste application, smoke or steam fumigation, ironing method, bian stone method, moxibustion, tuina therapy, cupping therapy, etc. in addition to intake of decoctions. The diversification of therapeutic means was also one of the signs of the improvement of medical level at that time. The discovery of the *Fifty-two Prescriptions*, which supplemented the medical contents of *Neijing* before, is a very precious medical heritage.

## 第十一节　藁城台西砭镰
### The Stone Scythe of Taixi Village, Gaocheng

藁城台西遗址中出土的类似镰刀的石质器物，其外缘弯曲钝圆，内缘锐利，长20厘米，最宽处5.4厘米，整体完整，仅柄端稍有磨损。石镰本来是农具，但经过专家分析鉴定，这件石镰，是一件割脓疮的手术刀，称为砭镰，是世界上现存最早的手术刀，距今3400多年。《山海经》中有关于砭镰的记载，表明了砭石是古代用来治病的一种工具。砭石包括石针、石砮、石镰，其大小不一，根据具体情况选用。其体积不宜过大，以单手使用方便为原则。类似用砭镰治疗疮痈方面的记载，从元、明一些医书中也可以找到。古代人常用砭镰切破肿疡、痈脓，排除瘀血和脓血，相当于现在外科手术刀。砭石疗法不断衍变创新，可用于疏通经络、调气活血、促进人体阴阳平衡，对一些疑难病、慢性病也有较好的治疗作用。秦汉时期，砭术与针、灸、药和导引按蹻并列为中医的五大医术。

Gaocheng Taixi Site unearthed a stone artifact shaped like a scythe whose outer edge was a curved blunt circle and inner edge sharp. It is 20 cm long. The widest part is of 5.4 cm. The whole is complete with only the handle slightly worn. A sickle was originally a farm tool, but after the experts' analysis and identification, this sickle turned out to be a scalpel to cut abscises, known as the stone scythe which is the earliest scalpel of more than 3400 years old. The records of bian stones in *The Classic of Mountains and Seas* show that bian stones were tools used in ancient times to cure diseases. They include stone needles, stone arrows, stone scythes with no certain standards of size, which are based on the specific situation and requirements of the disease. They should not be too large and used conveniently with one hand. Records about the treatment of carbuncle with scabbing can be found in some medical books of the Yuan and Ming Dynasties. In ancient times, stone scythes were commonly used to vent abscess to remove stasis, which is equivalent to the surgeon's scalpel now. The ancient people often used bian stones therapy for health care, which had a very good effect on dredging the meridians, activating qi and blood and promoting the balance of yin and yang in human body. It also had a better regulating effect on some difficult and chronic diseases. In the Qin and Han dynasties, acupuncture, moxibustion, medications and daoyin together with bian stones were listed as the five major medical skills of Chinese medicine.

考古文物 第九章

## 第十二节 《清明上河图》
### *Riverside Scene at Qingming Festival*

### 《清明上河图》——杨家应诊

*Riverside Scene at Qingming Festival* － Yang's Clinic

《清明上河图》中的一处门面前立有一块大招牌，上面写有"杨家应诊"四个字。可以推断，此处是一位姓杨的大夫开的诊所。门前站立一人，似乎在招呼前来就诊的人，服务之热情可见一斑。还有两人在大门外聊天，好像是大夫在送一位结束就医的病人，反复交代医嘱，病人有些依依不舍。右侧一位老者牵着一个孩童正在去就诊。前方一辆马车拉着一位病愈者急着赶路回家。画面生动形象，由于周边竞争激烈，主人不得不十分用心经营这家诊所。北宋时期，国家对中医的发展十分重视，专门成立负责药品制造和经营的官方机构，即熟药所，又称"卖药所"，从药材收购、检验、管理到监督中成药的制作，都有专人负责。后来，熟药所改名为医药惠民局，主要制造出售丸、散、膏、丹等中成药和药酒，这些药物服用简便、携带方便、易于保存，很受医生和病人欢迎。《清明上河图》中除了药铺，大街上还有一些摆摊设点叫卖膏药的人，这些场景直观反映了北宋城市的医疗状况，为后世研究提供了重要参考。

There is a store with a big sign standing in its front. Four words "Yang Jia Ying Zhen"are written above. It shows that this is a clinic run by a doctor whose surname is Yang. In front of the door stands a person who seems to greet the people who come to see a doctor. The enthusiasm of his service can be seen. Two other people are chatting away outside the gate. It seems that the doctor is sending a patient who has just seen a doctor here, repeatedly explaining the dose and method of medication, which makes the patient reluctant to leave. An elderly man on the right is towing a child to the clinic. A carriage is pulling a recovering man on his way home. The picture is vivid and rich in life flavor. Due to the fierce competition around, the owner has to run the clinic very carefully. During the Northern Song Dynasty, the state attached great importance to the development of traditional Chinese medicine. An official body, known as a pharmacy, was set up to manufacture and sell drugs. From the purchase, inspection and management of medicinal materials to the supervision of the production of proprietary Chinese medicines, there were special personnel in charge. Later, the institute was renamed Medical Relief Bureau, mainly manufacturing and selling pills, powder, paste, dan and other proprietary Chinese medicine and medicated liquor, which were easy to administer, carry and keep. They were very popular with doctors and patients. In addition to the clinics and pharmacies, the street was also full of people who had set up stalls selling poultices in *Riverside Scene at Qingming Festival*. These scenes directly reflect the medical conditions of the cities in the Northern Song Dynasty and provide an important reference for future studies.

考古文物 第九章

## 《清明上河图》——赵太丞家

*Riverside Scene at Qingming Festival* — Zhao Taicheng's Clinic

　　《清明上河图》中绘有多处药铺和诊所，其中描绘最详细的是画卷末端的"赵太丞家"。"太医丞"是宋代宫廷医官的名称。当时的东京开封是全国的药材集散地，上等的药铺大多由官宦人家或宫廷御医开设。这家药铺大概是赵姓医官所办，既是皇姓，又有官方背景，所在位置非常优越。"赵太丞家"门西有两块招牌，但字迹不清，其中一块有"五劳七伤"等字样，另一块像是"妇儿病不计利"之类的宣传语。中医所谓"五劳"指肝、心、脾、肺、肾五脏劳损；"七伤"指"大饱伤脾，大怒气逆伤肝，强力举重、久坐湿地伤肾，形寒饮冷伤肺，忧愁思虑伤心，风雨寒暑伤形，恐惧不节伤志"。从这些宣传语可以看出，这位"赵太丞"擅长内科、儿科、妇科，而且"妇儿病不计利"，可谓杏林春暖、医德高尚。屋内坐着一位中年妇女，怀抱小儿。二人面前立着一位长者，正低头审视着妇女怀中的小儿。可见"赵太丞家"不仅制售药品，还有医生坐堂诊病。画中给小儿看病的场景，可谓逼真生动。

　　There are many pharmacies and clinics in *Riverside Scene at Qingming Festival*, among which the most detailed one is "Zhao

Taicheng's Clinic" at the end of the scroll. Taiyicheng was the name of the imperial medical officer in the Song Dynasty. At that time, Kaifeng in Dongjing was the national medicinal material distribution center, where most of the first-class pharmacies were opened by the officials or court doctors. It was probably run by a medical officer surnamed Zhao, who had both a royal family name and an official background, so it was in a very good trade position. There are two signboards on the west door of the clinic, but the handwriting was not clear. One had "seven injuries due to excessive consumption of five zang-organs" and the like. The other one seemed to be the slogan about "making no profits from sick women or children". The so-called "wu lao" in Chinese medicine refers to the strain of the heart, liver, spleen, lungs and kidney. "Seven injuries" refers to "fullness in one's stomach damaging the spleen, rage damaging the liver, weight lifting and sitting in wetlands for long damaging the kidney, feeling cold and preference of cold drink damaging the lung, sorrow and worry damaging the heart, wind, rain, cold and heat damaging the body, fear and lack of self-discipline damaging one's determination". From the advertising, Doctor Zhao seemed to be good at internal medicine, pediatrics, gynecology and showed special benevolence to women and children which manifests noble medical ethics. Inside the house sat a middle-aged woman, holding a child in her arms. In front of them stood an elderly man, looking down at the child. It can be seen that "Zhao Taicheng's Clinic" not only produces and sells medicines, but also makes diagnosis and treatment. The scene of seeing a doctor in the picture is vivid.

# 古代神医及名医
## Ancient Divine Doctors and Famous Doctors

## 第一节 神 农
### Shennong

　　神农（公元前3245年－公元前3080年），即炎帝，生于历山（今湖北随州市境内），中国远古传说中的太阳神。神农姓姜，号神农氏，上古人物，有文字记载是在战国以后。他被世人尊称为"药祖""五谷先帝""神农大帝""地皇"等，是华夏太古三皇之一。传说神农是农业和医药的发明者。他教人医疗与农耕，因为他掌管医药及农业的神职，保佑农业收成、人民健康，所以被医馆、药行视为守护神。传说神农氏样貌奇特，人身牛首，三岁时便知稼穑，长大后身高八尺七寸，有龙颜大唇，身材瘦削，身体除四肢和脑袋外，都是透明的。传说神农氏尝尽百草，每服下有毒的药草后，他的内脏就会呈现黑色，因此什么药草对于人体哪个部位有影响就可以轻易地知道了，由于服下太多种毒药，积毒太深，又中了断肠草之毒，不幸身亡了。这些都是后世传说，说明他和黄帝一样，是中华民族文明之祖。

Shennong (3245 B.C. － 3080 B.C.), also known as Emperor Yan, was born in Lishan (now in Suizhou city, Hubei Province), the sun god in ancient Chinese legends. His surname is Jiang, also known as Shennongshi. Written records about him can be traced back to the Warring States Period. He is known as the "ancestor of medicine", "the first emperor of grain", "the emperor of earth" and so on. Legend has it that he is one of the three emperors of ancient Chinese mythology, the legendary inventor of agriculture and medicine. He taught people to use medicine and guarded agricultural harvest and the people's health. He is regarded as the patron saint by later hospitals and pharmacies. Shennong has the body of a man and the head of a cow, an image of semi-human and sei-animal. When he was three years old, he knew farming. When he grew up, he was eight chi seven cun (approximately 2.87 meters) tall with large lips and a thin figure. His body was transparent except for his limbs and head. Shennong tasted all kinds of herbs. As long as the herb was poisonous, his internal organs turned black after he swallowed it. Therefore, people learned to know which herb affected which part of the human body. Later, because he took in too many kinds of poisons that were accumulated in his body, he fell victim to the poison of deadly grass and died. These legends are deification of Emperor Yan from posterity to their ancestors. He is regarded as the ancestor of the Chinese civilization together with Yellow Emperor.

# 第二节　伊　尹
## Yi Yin

伊尹是商初重臣之一，尹为官名（相当于宰相）。他用烹调五味作引子，分析天下大势与为政之道，劝汤承担灭夏大任。汤了解到伊尹有经天纬地之才，便免其奴隶身份，授予他右相的职位，让他成了最高执政大臣。伊尹辅佐商汤，灭了夏朝最后一名君主——残暴的夏桀，建立了商朝。殷墟甲骨文中有关于后代祭祀伊尹的内容。甲骨文是巫师主持祭祀鬼神，占卜吉凶所用，其中甲骨文记载的疾病有20多种，虽然不能说与伊尹有直接关系，但伊尹肯定参与过类似的占卜活动。根据学者考证，伊尹在商朝的身份除了宰相外，还有一个更为重要的身份——巫师。商是一个非常崇信鬼神的朝代，国家大事小情都要通过占卜，因此巫师拥有崇高的地位。上古巫、史、医合一，巫师本身多兼有医者的功能。在医药方面，伊尹擅长经方。古代不少学者都认为，《汤液经法》是伊尹所撰写的。后人还认为中药汤剂也是伊尹所创。

Yi Yin was one of the most important ministers in the early Shang Dynasty. Yin was the official name (equivalent to the prime minister). He was born as a slave and cooked for the King Tang. Inspired by the relationship of five flavors in cooking, he recognized the general trend of the world and the way to govern it. He advised Tang to assume the responsibility of overthrowing Xia Jie. Tang knew that Yi Yin was talented, so he forgave his slave status and ordered him to be the chief prime minister and became the highest ruling minister. Yi Yin assisted Shang Tang in establishing the Shang Dynasty by destroying the tyrannical Jie, the last emperor of the Xia Dynasty. The inscriptions on bones and tortoise shells in the Ruins of Yin left by the Shang Dynasty have the contents of offering sacrifices to Yi Yin. Oracle-bone inscriptions were made by witches who offered sacrifices to the gods and goddesses for telling a fortune. Among them, there were about twenty kinds of diseases recorded on oracle-bone scripts. Although they were not directly related to Yi Yin, he must have participated in similar divination activities. According to scholars' research, Yi Yin's position in the Shang Dynasty was not only a minister in the regime, but also a sorcerer. Shang was a dynasty in which people believed in ghosts and spirits very much. All of the national affairs were solved through divination, so the sorcerer had a high status. In ancient times, witches also served for medical purpose. Yi Yin was good at prescriptions. Moreover, many scholars believed that Yi Yin wrote the *Classics of Decoctions*. Later generations also believed that the traditional Chinese medicine decoction was also created by Yi Yin.

## 伊尹与"汤液"的发明

Yi Yin and the Invention of Herbal Decoctions

　　伊尹，夏末商初人，他拥有高超的烹饪技巧，并在宰相位置上成绩卓著。最初他只是一个奴隶，专职为汤王做饭。伊尹对国事治理有自己鲜明的见解，他认为治大国如烹小鲜。语言虽简单，但哲理深刻，耐人寻味。有一次，伊尹见汤询问饭菜的事，说："做菜既不能太咸，也不能太淡，要调好佐料才行。治国如同做菜，既不能操之过急，也不能松弛懈怠，只有恰到好处，才能把事情办好。"商汤听了，很受启发，也看出伊尹才智出众，富有创见，便产生重用伊尹之意，于是汤王大胆地任命伊尹为宰相。由于他在烹饪和治国方面成绩卓著，使得人们往往忽视了他在医药方面的贡献，以至于他发明"汤液"的事鲜为人知。汤液是他在烹饪过程中摸索出来的，他认为生米、生菜能做成美味佳肴，营养丰富，口感上乘，那么将草药混合起来慢煮煎成汤液，更易发挥药效。经过反复实践，发明了草药汤液，此方法沿用至今。

In ancient times, there was a person who made outstanding achievements in the position of the prime minister and excellently skillful in cooking. His name was Yi Yin, born in the late Xia and early Shang Dynasties. At first, he was just a slave and worked exclusively as a cook for the King of Tang. Yi Yin had his own distinct views on governing a large country. He thought that governing a large country was like cooking a small fish. The description is simple but full of profound philosophy. Once Tang asked him about a meal. Yi Yin said, "The proper cooking is neither too salty nor too bland. You must adjust the ingredients well. Running a country is like cooking. You should neither rush it nor slack off. Only when it is just right can you get things right." When Shang Tang heard of this, he was very inspired. Knowing Yi Yin's outstanding intelligence and creativity, he had the idea of putting him in a higher position. As we expect, he boldly appointed him as the prime minister. Because of his remarkable achievements in cooking and governing, people tend to overlook his contributions to medicine. Little is known about the herbal decoctions he invented. This is what he found out from cooking. He thought raw rice and vegetable could be delicious, nutritious and tasty, so herbs could be more effective when they were slowly cooked into a decoction. After his repeated practice, herbal decoction was invented in this way, and this method is still used today.

## 第三节　扁　鹊
### Bian Que

　　扁鹊在中国医学史上是一个非常重要的人物。很多古籍都载有"扁鹊"的事迹。扁鹊对中医学的伟大贡献，从司马迁《史记》中可见一斑。然而由于年代久远，关于扁鹊是个体，还是群体以及其活动的年代，历来众说纷纭。其中，以西汉司马迁的观点最具代表性。司马迁认为，扁鹊姓"秦"、名"越人"，他在赵行医的时候，被称为"扁鹊"。隋唐时期有种说法认为，黄帝时代有一位神医"扁鹊"，因为秦越人的医术名冠当代，与轩辕时"扁鹊"的医术不相上下，所以当时的人称秦越人为"扁鹊"。还有一种观点认为，"扁鹊"为周秦时期良医的代名词。一些学者根据史料记载认为，扁鹊的事迹分别涉及赵简子、齐桓公、秦武王等人物，而这些人物各自所处的年代前后相去几百年，显然扁鹊的寿命是不可能有那么长的，因此认定"扁鹊"只是周秦良医的一种通称而已。"扁鹊"不是指某一个人，而是对周秦之间所有医术高超医生的一种称谓。不管事实如何，有一点是可以肯定的，扁鹊学派擅长脉诊，因此被后世誉为"脉学之宗"。

　　Bian Que is a very important person in the history of Chinese medicine. Many ancient books tell his stories. Bian Que's great contribution to traditional Chinese medicine can be proven from

Sima Qian's *Records of Historian*. However, due to its long history, there have been many opinions on whether Bian Que was an individual or a group of people and opinions varied as to the time of his existence. The view of Sima Qian in the Western Han Dynasty is the most important representative. Sima Qian believed that Bian Que had the surname "Qin" and the given name "Yueren". When he practiced medicine in Zhao State, he was called "Bian Que". There is a saying in the Sui and Tang Dynasties that there was a magic doctor named "Bian Que" in the Yellow Emperor's time. Because the name of the Qin Yueren's medical skill was equal to that of "Bian Que" in Xuanyuan era, people called Qin Yueren "Bian Que". There is another view that "Bian Que" was the common name of good doctors between the Zhou and Qin Dynasties. Some scholars had recorded the deeds of Bian Que in historical records, including Zhao Jianzi, Marquis Huan of Qi State, King Wu of Qin, etc. The times in which these characters lived have a span of several hundred years while it is obvious that Bian Que's life is not that long. Therefore, Bian Que is regarded as a general name for the excellent doctors of Zhou and Qin Dynasties. "Bian Que" is not a person, but a name for all the highly skilled doctors between Zhou and Qin. No matter what the facts are, one thing is certain: Bian Que School is good at pulse diagnosis, so it is praised as "the origin of pulse" by later generations.

## 扁鹊三兄弟

Bian Que and His Two Brothers

扁鹊云游各国，为君侯们看病，也为百姓们解除疾患，因而名扬天下。有一次，魏文王问名医扁鹊，"你们家兄弟三人，都精于医术，谁是医术最好的呢？"扁鹊说："大哥最好，二哥差些，我是三人中最差的一个。"魏文王不解地问："为什么？"扁鹊解释说："大哥治病，是在病情发作之前，那时候病人自己还不觉得有病，但大哥就下药铲除了病根。他的医术不被人知晓，所以没有名气，只是在我们家中被推崇备至。我的二哥治病，是在病刚开始发作的时候，症状尚不十分明显，病人也没有觉得痛苦，二哥就能药到病除。于是，乡里人都认为二哥只是治小病很灵。我治病，都是在病情十分严重的时候，病人痛苦万分，病人的家属心急如焚。此时，他们看到我在穴位上针刺，用针放血，或在患处敷以毒药以毒攻毒，或动大手术直指病灶，使病情得到缓解或很快治愈，我名闻天下便因为此罢了。"魏文王大悟。就整个社会人群的生存发展而言，人们不仅需要像扁鹊那样高效率治已病的良医，更需要众多治未病、治欲病的上医、中医。

When Bian Que traveled in different states, he treated diseases for both the kings and the common people. So he became famous. Once, the King Wen of Wei asked Bian Que, "You three brothers are all skilled in medicine. Who is the best?" Bian Que answered, "My eldest brother is the best, the second brother is better. I am the worst of the three." The King Wen of Wei asked, "Why?" Bian Que explained, "The eldest brother treated the disease before its onset when the patient himself did not feel sick, but he prescribed medicine to eradicate the root of the disease, making his medical skills difficult to be recognized, so he is not famous, but in our family he is highly respected. My second elder brother treated the disease at its beginning. The symptoms were not very obvious and the patient did not feel painful. The villagers regard him as an ordinary doctor who could only treat some minor illnesses because of his little reputation. I treated the patient under a very serious condition, who was in great pain and whose family was very anxious. At this point, they saw me pierce the acupoints and bleed with the needle, or put a drastic medicine on the lesion to cure an emergency, or perform a major operation directly on the focus of the disease so that the patient's condition could be alleviated or quickly cured, That's why I'm famous." The King Wen of Wei was enlightened. In terms of the survival and development of the whole social population, people not only need skillful doctors like Bian Que to treat the serious disease, but also need a large number of superior and medium doctors who are good at preventive treatment or treatment based on light symptoms.

## 扁鹊——病有六不治

### Even Bian Que Can't Cure You!

春秋战国时期名医扁鹊，有"病有六不治"之说。骄恣不论于理，一不治也。轻身重财，二不治也。衣食不能适，三不治也。阴阳并，藏气不定，四不治也。形羸不能服药，五不治也。信巫不信医，六不治也。即不治不讲道理、不遵医嘱的人，他们把医生的话当成耳旁风，不按时服药，消极地对抗治疗；不治只重视钱财而不重视养生的人，他们把钱财看得比自己生命还重要；不治过于挑剔的人，良药可以根除疾病，但无法根除恶习；不治体内气血错乱、脏腑功能严重衰竭的人，这种人已经病入膏肓，错过了最佳治疗时间；不治身体极度羸弱、不能服药或不能承受药力的人；不治只相信鬼神、不信任医学的人，这种人即便勉强接受医疗，也会走旁门左道。扁鹊在医学实践道路上抛弃巫术，以自己精湛的医术，开启了医学之路。扁鹊的"六不治"，告诫人们不要把自己陷入这六种情况。毕竟医患关系需要通过双方的努力才能够得到很好的维护。

Bian Que, a famous doctor in the Spring and Autumn Period and Warring States Period, said that "he couldn't cure six kinds of patients". The first kind refers to arrogant, unhearing or ungovernable people. Those who do not follow the doctor's advice but take the doctor's words as wind and do not take medicine on time. They react negatively to therapy. The second kind of patients worship money but ignore health. They value money more than their own life. The third patients are too critical of food and clothing. Good medicine can root out diseases, but not bad habits. The fourth kind of patients with disorder of qi and blood and serious failure of zang-fu organs are so ill that they miss the best time for treatment. The fifth kind of patients are so weak that they are unable to take or withstand the effects of medications. The sixth group of patients only believe in ghosts and detest medicine. Such people will go astray even if they grudgingly accept medical treatment. Bian Que abandoned witchcraft on the road of medical practice. With his excellent medical skills, he opened the road of ancient Chinese medicine and broke through the fog and interference of witchcraft and superstition. Bian Que's "difficulty in treating the six kinds of patients" warned people of avoiding themselves into these six situations. After all, the doctor-patient relationship can only be well maintained through the efforts of both sides.

# 第四节 仓 公
## Cang Gong

《史记·扁鹊仓公列传》是一篇记叙古代名医事迹的合传。一位是战国时期的扁鹊，另一位是西汉初年的淳于意。仓公，是齐国都城管理粮仓的长官，姓淳于名叫意（约公元前205 - ？）。淳于意创立了诊籍，即病历。司马迁在《史记·扁鹊仓公列传》中详尽地记录了淳于意的这些病历，内容包括姓名、年龄、性别、职业、籍里、病名、脉象、病状、诊断、病因、治疗、疗效、预后等，从中反映了淳于意的医疗学术思想与医案记录上的创造性贡献。这是我国医学史上最早见于史书记载的病案记录，为我们留下了研究汉代医学的宝贵史料。这些病历涉及了现代医学的消化科、泌尿科、呼吸科、心血管科、内分泌科、脑血管科、传染病科、外科、妇产科、儿科等。难能可贵的是，在25个病历中，既有成功的经验，也有失败的教训，对于没有治好的病历并不加以粉饰和掩盖。这种实事求是、恭敬严谨的态度正是医者学习的楷模。淳于意针对病人的病情，不仅仅采用药物治疗，还广泛运用各种物理疗法及针灸疗法。

*The Biography of Bian Que and Cang Gong of Records of Historian* records the deeds of some famous doctors in ancient times. One is Bian Que in the Warring States Period and the other is

Chunyu Yi in the early Western Han Dynasty. Cang Gong was the chief granary officer in the capital of the state of Qi. His surname was Chunyu and his first name was Yi (c. 205 B.C － ?). Chunyu Yi created medical records. Sima Qian recorded these medical records in detail in his *Records of Historian*. They include patients' names, ages, sexes, occupations, history, names of diseases, pulses, symptoms, diagnosis, etiology, treatment, curative effects, prognosis, etc., which reflect his sincere medical academic thoughts and creative contribution in the medical records. These are the earliest medical records in the history of Chinese medicine, leaving us precious historical materials for studying medicine in the Han Dynasty. These cases involve digestive, urinary, respiratory, cardiovascular, endocrine, cerebrovascular and infectious diseases as well as surgery, obstetrics and gynecology, pediatrics of modern medicine, which have significance for research. What is remarkable is that there are both successful experiences and failures in the 25 cases with no glossing over or covering up the cases that had not been cured. This practical, respectful and rigorous attitude is a model for doctors to learn from. Chunyu Yi used drugs, physical therapies and acupuncture to treat patients' conditions.

## 第五节　华　佗
### Hua Tuo

　　华佗（约145年－208年），汉末沛国谯县（今安徽亳州）人，东汉末年医学家，与董奉、张仲景并称为"建安三神医"。华佗曾在外游学，行医的足迹遍及了安徽、河南、山东、江苏等地。华佗精通内、外、妇、儿、五官各科，尤其擅长外科，精于手术，被尊称为"外科鼻祖"。华佗不仅医术高明，还有高贵的品德。他不图名利，不求仕途，宁愿做一个四处奔波，治病救人的民间医生。据《后汉书》记载，华佗用针灸治好了曹操久治不愈的头痛病，曹操曾多次要求华佗留在身边做侍医，华佗以妻子生病为由返乡。曹操就将华佗逮捕治罪，华佗仍然拒不从命。华佗预料到会遭不幸，就将携带的医书一卷交给狱卒，希望能保存下来流传后世，造福百姓。但狱卒怕受连累，不敢收下。华佗非常失望，一怒之下，将医书付之一炬。最后，华佗不幸被曹操杀害，他的医书也就此失传。后人多用神医华佗称呼他，又以"华佗再世""元化重生"称誉医术杰出的医师。

　　Hua Tuo (about 145 A.D. － 208 A.D.), a physician at the end of the Eastern Han Dynasty, was born at Qiao county in Peiguo (now Bozhou, Anhui Province). He and Dong Feng, Zhang Zhongjing were known as the "Three Magic Doctors in Jian'an Period". When he was young, he studied and practiced medicine in Anhui, Henan, Shandong, Jiangsu and other places. He did not seek the official career. With comprehensive medical skills, he was proficient in internal and external medicine, as well as women, children, ENT, acupuncture and moxibustion departments. He was especially good at surgery, known as the "forefather of surgery" in China. Hua Tuo was not only skillful in medicine, but also of noble morality. Instead of seeking fame and wealth, he would rather be a folk doctor running around, treating patients and saving people than be an official in the court. According to *The Book of Later Han*, Hua Tuo used acupuncture to cure Cao Cao's headache. Cao repeatedly asked Hua to stay with him as a private doctor. Hua refused and returned home on the grounds that his wife was ill. Later, Cao Cao arrested Hua Tuo and sentenced him to death, but Hua Tuo still refused to obey. Anticipating his misfortune, Hua Tuo handed his medical book to the jailer in the hope that it would be preserved and handed down for the benefit of the people. But the jailer did not dare to take it for fear of being harmed. Hua Tuo was so disappointed that he set the medical books on fire in anger. At last, Hua Tuo was killed by Cao Cao and his medical book was lost. Later, people praise the physicians who have outstanding medical skills as "Reborn Hua Tuo".

## 第六节　董　奉
**Dong Feng**

　　董奉，字君异，东汉末年东吴侯官（今福建长乐）人。史料考证，董奉出生于169年，204年离家行医，经过几年医学实践，他名声大振。东汉末年，朝廷腐败，外戚专权，战事不断，加之水旱蝗灾连年不绝、疫病流行，民不聊生。董奉在交州一带行医的时候，恰遇交州太守病危。董奉将3粒药丸放入病人口中，用水送下。稍后，病人手足能动，肤色逐渐转好，半日后即能坐起，4日后能说话，不久病愈。董奉住在太守府中之时，恰逢太守阴谋反叛朝廷，主人担心董奉泄漏消息，想要加害董奉。董奉利用气功装死，骗过太守后逃走。207年左右，董奉隐居庐山。其间，他一面练功，一面行医。董奉医术高明，治病不取钱物，只要求重病愈者在山中栽杏5株，轻病愈者栽杏1株。数年之后，杏树郁然成林。春天杏子成熟的时候，董奉便在树下建一间草屋来储藏杏子。需要杏子的人，可用谷子交换。董奉再将所得的谷子赈济贫民。董奉施医济世，开创了人与自然生态和谐共荣的杏林园。

　　Dong Feng, courtesy name Jun Yi, was a man of Houguan (now Changle, Fujian) in the late Eastern Han Dynasty. According to historical records, Dong was born in 169 A.D. and left home in 204 A.D. to practice medicine. After several years, he made a reputation for himself. At the end of the Eastern Han Dynasty, the court was corrupt. The empress's relatives had the exclusive power with wars continuing year after year. Floods, droughts, locust plague and epidemic diseases were incessant. Miserable people were living in poverty. When Dong Feng was practicing medicine in the region of Jiaozhou, he happened to meet the governor critically ill who was on his deathbed for three days. Dong put three pills into the patient's mouth and poured water down them. Later, the patient could move his hands and feet. His skin color gradually changed to life. He was able to sit up after half a day and he could speak four days later. He recovered soon. At that time Dong Feng lived in the governor's house. Later, the governor plotted to rebel against the imperial court. He was afraid that Dong Feng would reveal his plot and wanted to kill him. Dong Bong pretended to be dead with qigong and fled later. Dong Feng, fearing that something might happen to him, was forced to choose Mount Lu as his retreat around 207 A.D.. At Mount Lu, he practiced medicine while practicing qigong. Dong Feng was a skilled doctor. He did not take money to cure diseases, but required the seriously ill to plant 5 apricot trees in the mountains after his recovery and the mild patient 1 apricot tree. A few years later, there were ten thousand apricot trees, blossoming into a forest. In the spring, when the apricots were ripe, Dong built a hut under the tree to store the apricots. Those who wanted apricots could exchange them with corn. He gave food to the needy and gave it to them on the way. Dong Feng pursued medicine and helped the diseased. He created the apricot forest, in which human beings and nature coexist harmoniously.

# 第七节　张仲景
## Zhang Zhongjing

张仲景，名机，字仲景，东汉南阳涅阳县（今河南省邓州市穰东镇张寨村）人，东汉末年著名医学家，被后人尊称为医圣。史书记载，东汉末年战争频繁，加上自然灾害，导致了一种叫"伤寒"的疫病流行。这种病传染性强，致死率高。东汉桓帝时大疫三次，灵帝时大疫五次，献帝建安年间疫病流行更甚。成千上万的人被病魔吞噬，以致造成了十室九空的景象。建安年间，张仲景行医游历各地，目睹了疫病流行对百姓造成的严重后果，他痛下决心，潜心研究伤寒病的诊治方法，一定要制服伤寒这个瘟神。为此，张仲景广泛收集医方，经过数十年的努力，写成了传世巨著《伤寒杂病论》，确立的辨证论治原则，是中医临床的基本原则，是中医的灵魂所在。张仲景是我国历史上最杰出的医学家之一，为我国的医学发展做出了重要的贡献。到了晋代，名医王叔和对《伤寒杂病论》进行了整理。到了宋代，才逐渐分为《伤寒论》《金匮要略》。

Zhang Zhongjing whose first name was Ji and courtesy name was Zhongjing, was born in Niyang County, Nanyang in the Eastern Han Dynasty (present-day Zhangzhai Village, Zhongdong Town, Dengzhou City, Henan Province). He was a famous medical expert in the late Eastern Han Dynasty, and was honored as the medical saint by later generations. According to historical records, wars and natural disasters in the late Eastern Han Dynasty caused an epidemic of typhoid fever which was highly contagious and lethal frequently happened. In the Eastern Han Dynasty, there were three severe epidemics during Emperor Huan's reign and five epidemics during Emperor Ling's reign, even seriously during Emperor Xian's reign. Tens of thousands of people were engulfed by the epidemics, resulting in an unprecedented disaster. During the Jian'an Period, Zhang Zhongjing practiced medicine in the country, witnessing with his own eyes the serious consequences of various epidemics on the grassroots. He resolved to devote himself to the diagnosis and treatment of typhoid fever and to subdue the pestilence. In this regard, Zhang Zhongjing extensively collected medical prescriptions. After decades of painstaking efforts, he wrote a masterpiece "*On Typhoid Fever and Miscellaneous Diseases*". The principle of treatment based on syndrome differentiation established by it is the basic principle of TCM clinical practice and the essence of TCM. Zhang Zhongjing is one of the most outstanding doctors in China's history. He has made important contributions to the development of Chinese medicine. In the Jin Dynasty, the famous doctor Wang Shuhe tried to sort out his manuscripts. In the Song Dynasty, it was gradually divided into two books, namely, *Treatise on Febrile Diseases* and *Synopsis of The Golden Chamber*.

## 张仲景——辨证论治

## Zhang Zhongjing － Treatment Based on Syndrome Differentiation

张仲景受人敬仰的重要原因之一，是他的《伤寒杂病论》体现出来的"辨证论治"的重要医学思想，它的出现对后世中医学发展起到了重要的影响作用。使用寒凉药物治疗热性病是中医的"正治法"，而使用温热的药物治疗热性病属于"反治法"。这两种截然不同的治疗方法都是用于治疗热性疾病的，相同的症状不同的治疗方法，如何区别和选择呢？这就要辨证。不能只看表面症状，医生还要通过望闻问切和辨证分析，得出证候特点，才能给处方。这种"透过现象看本质"的诊断方法，就是著名的"辨证论治"观点。这也是几千年来中医长盛不衰，至今仍能傲立于世界医林的"拿手绝活儿"。同时，书中提出了治疗外感病的一种重要的分类方法，就是将病邪由浅入深地分为6个阶段，每个阶段都有一些共同的症状特点并衍生出很多变化，这一阶段的用方和选药就可以局限在某一范围，只要辨证准确，方子运用得当就会有很好的疗效，这种方法后人称为"六经辨证"。

One of the important reasons for Zhang Zhongjing's being admired is the important medical thought of "treatment based on syndrome differentiation" embodied in his *Treatise on Cold Damage and Miscellaneous Diseases.* Its appearance played a dominant role in the development of Chinese medicine in later generations. The use of cold and cool drugs to treat the heat syndrome is the "treatment based on cause of disease" while the use of warm drugs to treat them is known as "treatment based on similar property of symptoms and drugs". But these two very different treatments are used to treat diseases of the same properties. That is to say, they share the same symptoms but with different treatments. How to distinguish between them and choose one? Differentiation. Doctors should not only learn about the symptoms, but also the characteristics of syndromes through observation, smelling and listening, questioning and pulse-taking as well as syndrome analysis so as to give prescriptions. This diagnostic method of "to see the essence from the phenomenon" is known as "syndrome differentiation for treatment" which is the reason why traditional Chinese medicine has flourished for thousands of years in the world till now. At the same time, an important classification method for the treatment of exogenous diseases is proposed in the book, which is to divide the pathogenic factors into six stages from shallow to deep locations. Each stage has some common symptomatic characteristics and many variations, during which the prescription and drug selection could be limited to a certain range. As long as the syndrome differentiation is accurate, the application of prescription will have a good curative effect. This method is later called "treatment based on differentiation of symptoms and signs of the six meridians".

## 张仲景——《伤寒杂病论》（一）

*Zhang Zhongjing － On Cold Damage and Miscellaneous Diseases* (I)

张仲景的《伤寒杂病论》集秦汉以来医药理论之大成，被广泛应用于医疗实践，是我国医学史上影响力最大的古代医著之一，也是我国第一部临床治疗学方面的巨著。《伤寒杂病论》的贡献，首先在于它确立了中医辨证论治的基本法则。对于治则和方药，《伤寒杂病论》的贡献也十分突出。书中提出的治则以整体观念为指导，调整阴阳，扶正祛邪，还有汗、吐、下、和、温、清、消、补诸法，并在此基础上创立了一系列疗效确切的方剂。据统计，《伤寒论》载方113个，《金匮要略》载方262个，除去重复部分，两书实收方剂269个。另外，在剂型上此书也勇于创新，其类型之多，已大大超过了汉代以前的各种方书，有汤剂、丸剂、散剂、膏剂、酒剂、洗剂、浴剂、熏剂、滴耳剂、灌鼻剂、吹鼻剂、灌肠剂、阴道栓剂、肛门栓剂等。此外，对各种剂型制法的记载也十分详细，尤其是汤剂的煎法、服法。所以后世称张仲景的《伤寒杂病论》为"方书之祖"，称该书所列方剂为"经方"。

*Treatise on Cold Damage and Miscellaneous Diseases* by Zhang Zhongjing has been a collection of medical theories since the Qin and Han Dynasties and widely used in medical practice.

It is one of the most influential classical medical works in the history of Chinese medicine and also the first great work in clinical therapeutics. It makes contributions to the development and establishment of the basic principle of treatment based on syndrome differentiation of TCM. For the treatment and prescriptions, its contribution is also very prominent. Guided by the holistic concept, the therapeutic principles in the book include the adjustment of yin and yang, strengthening the vital qi and eliminating the pathogenic factors, as well as the methods of sweating, vomiting, discharging, regulating, warming, resolving, eliminating and tonifying. On this basis, a series of effective prescriptions are created. According to statistics, *Treatise on Cold Damage* contains 113 prescriptions and *Synopsis of the Golden Chamber* contains 262 prescriptions. In addition, this book also has the courage to innovate on the dosage forms, and its variety is so numerous that it has greatly exceeded all kinds of previous prescriptions before the Han Dynasty. There are such dosage forms as decoction, pill, powder, cream, liquor, lotion, bath, fumigant, ear drops, nasal irrigation, nasal blowing, enema, vaginal suppository, anal suppository and so on. In addition, the preparation methods of various dosage forms are recorded in great detail and the decoctions and dosages are also explained in great detail. Therefore, Zhang Zhongjing's *Treatise on Cold Damage and Miscellaneous Diseases* is later called the "ancestor of prescriptions books", and the prescriptions listed in the book are called "Prescription Classics".

## 张仲景——《伤寒杂病论》（二）

### Zhang Zhongjing — *Treatise on Cold Damage and Miscellaneous Diseases*（Ⅱ）

公元205年，张仲景所著的《伤寒杂病论》对推动后世医学的发展起了巨大的作用。该书对针刺、灸烙、温熨、药摩、吹耳等治疗方法有诸多阐述；另外，对许多急救方法也有收集，如自缢、食物中毒等病人有独特的救治方法。其中对自缢的救治，类似现代的人工呼吸。这些都是祖国医学中的宝贵资料。《伤寒杂病论》奠定了张仲景在中医学史上的重要地位，并且随着时间的推移，这部专著的科学价值得以显露，成为后世医者必读的重要医籍。张仲景因其对医学的杰出贡献被后人称为"医圣"。后来，该书流传海外，同样受到国外医学界的推崇，成为海外医疗人士研读的重要典籍。据不完全统计，自晋代至今，整理、注释、研究《伤寒杂病论》的中外学者超过千家。邻国日本自康平年间（相当于我国宋朝）以来，研究《伤寒论》的学者也有近200家。此外，朝鲜、越南、印度尼西亚、新加坡、蒙古等国的医学发展也都不同程度地受到此书的影响。

The medical book *Treatise on Cold Damage and Miscellaneous Diseases* written by Zhang Zhongjing in 205 A.D. has played a great role in promoting the development of medicine in later generations.

For example, the therapeutic methods of acupuncture, moxibustion, hot ironing, medicated rubbing, ear blowing and so on are elaborated. In addition, many first aid methods are also collected, such as the treatments of hanging, food poisoning and so on are quite unique. Especially the manipulation of rescuing a hanging person is very similar to the modern artificial respiration. These are all valuable materials in Chinese medicine. *Treatise on Cold Damage and Miscellaneous Diseases* establishes Zhang Zhongjing's important position in the history of TCM and the scientific value of this monograph is more and more revealed with the passage of time. It has become an important medical book that all medical practitioners must read. Zhang Zhongjing is also known as the "medical saint" for his outstanding contributions to medicine. The book was spread abroad after its existence, also highly respected by the foreign medical community and became an important study of classical books. According to incomplete statistics, from the Jin Dynasty to now, there are more than a thousand Chinese and foreign scholars who have filed, annotated and studied it. Since the reign of Emperor Kangping in neighboring Japan (equivalent to the Song Dynasty in China), there have been nearly 200 scholars studying it. In addition, the medical development of Korea, Vietnam, Indonesia, Singapore, Mongolia and other countries are also affected and promoted by it to varying degrees.

古代神医及名医　第十章

## "堂"的来历

The History of "Tang"

在封建时代，做官的人不能随便进入民宅。可是不接触百姓，有官职的医生就不能为他们诊病。相传，张仲景当时官居长沙太守，仍心系治病救人，不忘百姓疾苦。他想了一个办法，每逢农历初一和十五，在后堂或自己家中给百姓治病。他让衙役贴出安民告示，告诉老百姓这一消息。他的举动在当地产生了强烈的反响，老百姓无不感激，再加上他一反封建官吏的官老爷作风，对前来求医的人总是热情接待，细心诊治，从不拒绝，老百姓便对张仲景更加拥戴。时间久了，形成了惯例。他的衙门前便聚集了来自各方求医看病的老百姓，甚至有远道而来的。正值疫疠流行，前来治病的人越来越多，使他应接不暇，于是他干脆把诊所搬到了大堂，坐堂应诊，首创了坐堂的先例。后来人们把坐在药铺里给人看病的医生，也称为"坐堂医生"，用来纪念张仲景。再后来人们给药铺取名时，往往在名字后面附上一个"堂"字，像现在北京的同仁堂、杭州的胡庆余堂等。

In feudal times and a society with strict class concept, officials were not closely connected to grassroots. But doctors couldn't treat patients without touching them. Zhang Zhongjing was then the prefect of Changsha. He was concerned with clinical practice and did not forget to relieve the sufferings of the common people. He had an idea of treating people in the back hall or in his own home. He had his men put up the placards to tell the people the news. His action had a strong effect on the local people, and they all applauded it. In addition to his anti-feudal officialdom, he was always hospitable to those who came for medical help. He made careful diagnosis and treatment and never refused anyone who came to see him. The common people were thankful and respectful to him. Over time, it had become a routine. On the 1st and 15th days of the lunar calendar, people gathered in front of his office to seek medical treatment. Some even came from afar with luggage. More and more people came to see Zhang Zhongjing when the epidemic was spreading, which kept him very busy. So he simply moved his clinic to the official lobby, which was the first example for a famous doctor to treat patients in the official place. Later, people called any doctor who sit in the pharmacy to treat patients "Zuotang Doctor" in memory of Zhang Zhongjing. And when people name a pharmacy, they often attach the character "Tang" to the name, such as "Tongren Hall" in Beijing and "Huqingyu Hall" in Hangzhou.

## 张仲景——祛寒娇耳汤

Zhang Zhongjing － Soup for Dispelling Cold

　　张仲景退休那年冬天，寒风刺骨，雪花纷飞。在河边，他看到无家可归的人面黄肌瘦，衣不遮体，因为寒冷，把耳朵都冻烂了，张仲景看到心里十分难受。于是，他研制了一个可以御寒的食疗方子，叫"祛寒娇耳汤"，就是把羊肉和一些祛寒的药物放在锅里煮，熟了以后捞出来切碎，用面皮包成耳朵的样子，再用原汤将包好馅料的面皮煮熟。面皮包好后，样子像耳朵，又因为目的是防止耳朵冻烂，所以张仲景给它取名叫"娇耳"。人们吃了"娇耳"，喝了汤，浑身发暖，两只耳朵热起来了，耳朵的冻伤自然就好了。据说张仲景是在冬至这天去世的，又是在冬至这天为大家舍"祛寒娇耳汤"的，为了纪念他，从此大家在冬至这天都吃一顿饺子。"祛寒娇耳汤"很少有人吃了，但大家在冬至这天吃饺子的习俗流传了下来。并且饺子的种类和形状也有了很大改进，有中国人的地方就有饺子，饺子也成了代表阖家团圆的食品，然而张仲景的名字和饺子的联系却很少有人再提到了。

　　It was a bitterly cold winter when Zhang Zhongjing retired. On the bank of the river, many homeless people were pale and thin with their bodies uncovered and their ears had frostbite due to exposure to the cold temperature. Zhang zhongjing felt very sympathetic. After some trials, he developed a diet prescription to keep out cold, called "Jiaoer Soup for Dispelling Cold". In fact, it is a mutton soup with some anti-cold medicine boiled in the pot. Then the cooked mutton was pulled out and chopped, which was wrapped in dough sheets and made into ear-shape dumplings, and then boil the dumplings in the pot with their original soup. Zhang Zhongjing named it "Jiaoer" because of its effect on preventing the ear from frostnip. The people ate the "Jiaoer" and drank the soup. Their bodies became warm all over and their ears became warm. No one suffered from frostbite any more. It is said that Zhang Zhongjing died on the day of the Winter Solstice and gave out the "Jiaoer Soup for Cold Dispelling " for everyone on that day. In order to commemorate him, people would make dumplings on the day of the Winter Solstice and they would not suffer from frostbite in winter. " Jiaoer Soup for Cold Dispelling" is rarely eaten by modern people, but the custom of eating dumplings on the day of Winter Solstice has been passed down. And the kinds and shapes of dumplings have been greatly evolved. Wherever there are Chinese people, there are dumplings, which has become a symbol of family reunion, but Zhang Zhongjing's name is rarely associated with dumplings later.

## 第八节　孙思邈
### Sun Simiao

　　孙思邈（约581－682年），唐代医学家，中医医德规范制定人，被尊为"药王"，京兆华原（今陕西耀州）人。隋大业（605－618年）时期，他游学四川，后隐于终南山，写了不少道家炼丹方面的著作。孙思邈在数十年的临床实践中，深感古代医方的散乱浩繁，难以检索，于是他博取群经，结合自己的临床经验，广泛收集民间流传的药方，编著成《千金要方》和《千金翼方》。唐高宗显庆四年（659年），他完成了世界上第一部国家药典《唐新本草》。《唐新本草》反映了唐初医学的发展水平。孙思邈通晓养生之术，虽年过百岁但视听不衰。他将儒家、道家以及古印度佛家的养生思想与中医学的养生理论相结合，提出了许多切实可行的养生方法。时至今日，这些方法也还在指导着人们的日常生活，如心态要保持平衡，不要一味追求名利；饮食应有所节制，不要暴饮暴食；气血应注意流通，不要懒惰呆滞不动；生活要起居有常，不要违反自然规律等。唐高宗上元元年（674年），孙思邈年高有病，返回故里。永淳元年（682年），与世长辞。

　　Sun Simiao (about 581 A.D. － 682 A.D.) was a medical practitioner in the Tang Dynasty who formulated the norms of medical ethics in traditional Chinese medicine and was respected as the "king of medicine". He was born in Huayuan (now Yao County, Shaanxi Province). During the reign of the Sui Daye (605 A.D. — 618 A.D.), he traveled to Sichuan to study alchemy, where he lived in the Zhongnan Mountain and wrote many works on Taoist alchemy. In his decades of clinical practice, Sun Simiao deeply felt the chaos and complexity of ancient medical prescriptions and their difficulty in consultation. Therefore, he learned from the classics, combined with his clinical experience, and extensively collected the folk prescriptions, and compiled them into *Qianjin Yaofang* and *Qianjin Yifang*. In 659, he completed the world's first national pharmacopoeia, *New Materia Medica of Tang Dynasty*, which reflected the development level of medicine in the early Tang Dynasty. Sun Simiao knew well how to maintain health and had retained his eyesight and hearing well beyond the age of 100. He absorbed the thoughts of Confucianism, Taoism, and Buddhism from ancient India into the theories of traditional Chinese medicine. Many of his practical ways of keeping fit are still guiding people's daily life today. For example, keep a balanced mind; do not blindly pursue fame and wealth; diet should be moderate; do not overeat; pay attention to the circulation of qi and blood, do not be lazy and dull; live regularly and don't violate the laws of nature, etc. In the first year of Emperor Gaozong of the Tang Dynasty (674 A.D.), Sun Simiao fell ill at an advanced age so he implored to return to his native land. In the first year of Yongchun (682 A.D.), he passed away.

## 《千金要方》

*Qianjin Yaofang*

《千金要方》又称《备急千金要方》《千金方》，是中国古代中医学经典著作之一，共30卷，是综合性临床医著，被誉为中国最早的临床百科全书，作者是唐朝孙思邈。《千金要方》总结了唐代以前医学成就，书中首篇《大医精诚》《大医习业》，是中医学伦理学的基础。其中，对妇科、儿科的论述，奠定了宋代妇科、儿科独立的基础。《千金要方》提倡以"五脏六腑为纲，寒热虚实为目"治内科病，并开创了脏腑分类方剂的先河。对针灸的论述，为针灸治疗准绳。阿是穴的选用、"同身寸"的提倡，对针灸取穴的准确性颇有帮助。《千金要方》对方剂学发展贡献也巨大，书中收集了从张仲景时代直至孙思邈的临床经验，历数百年的方剂成就，特别是源流各异的方剂用药，显示出孙思邈的博极医源和精湛医技。后人称《千金方》为方书之祖。《千金要方》在食疗、养生、养老方面也做出了巨大贡献。《千金要方》一书广闻博采，内容丰富，对我国古代医家，以及周边等国的医学发展的影响都非常大。

*Qianjin Yaofang*, also known as *Beiji Qianjin Yaofang* and *Qianjin Fang*, is one of the classic works of ancient TCM with a total of 30 volumes. It is a comprehensive medical work and is regarded as the earliest clinical encyclopedia in China. It was written by Sun Simiao in the Tang Dynasty and published in the third year of Yonghui. *Qianjin Yaofang* summarizes medical achievements before the Tang Dynasty. The first chapter of the book, "Great Medical Sincerity", "Great Medical Practice", is the basis of TCM ethics. Besides, the special treatises on gynecology and pediatrics lay the foundation for the division of gynecology and pediatrics in the Song Dynasty. It advocates the treatment of internal diseases with "the five zang-organs and six fu-organs as the outline and cold, heat and deficiency as the suborders", and pioneers the classification of the zang-fu organs. The discussion of indications based on acupoints provides the criterion for acupuncture and moxibustion treatment. The selection of Ashi acupoints and the promotion of "proportional unit of the middle finger" are of great help to the accuracy of acupuncture point selection. *Qianjin Yaofang* contributes a lot to the development of formulology. The clinical experience from Zhang Zhongjing to Sun Simiao, the prescriptions of hundreds of years, especially those of different sources and schools, are collected in the book which shows Sun Simiao's brilliant and exquisite medical skills. *Qianjin Fang* is honored as the founder of prescriptions. It has also made great contributions to diet therapy, health care and elderly caring. With rich contents, the classic work is widely read. It has a great impact on the medical development in ancient China as well as surrounding countries.

## 孙思邈——悬丝诊脉

## Sun Simiao － Feeling the Pulse with a Thread

相传，唐贞观年间，太宗李世民的长孙皇后怀孕已十多个月却不能分娩。虽然经过不少太医医治，但病情一直不见好转。唐太宗便派遣使臣星夜将孙思邈召进了皇宫。在封建社会，由于有"男女授受不亲"的礼教思想束缚，医生给宫内妃嫔看病，大都不能靠近身边，只能根据旁人的口述，开出诊治处方。孙思邈就叫来了皇后身边的宫女细问病情，并对太医的病历处方认真审阅，基本掌握了皇后的病情。然后，他取出一条红线，叫宫女把线系在皇后手腕上，另一端从竹帘拉出来，孙思邈捏着，在皇后房外开始"引线诊脉"。孙思邈诊断完毕，向太宗禀告了病因并请皇后左手扶着竹帘，孙思邈看准穴位猛扎了一针，皇后疼痛，浑身一颤抖。不一会儿，只听得婴儿呱呱啼哭之声，皇后产下了皇子，人也苏醒了！太宗大喜，请孙思邈入朝为官，但是他立志漂泊四方为广大百姓治病，婉言谢绝了太宗赐给的官位。之后，撰写了《千金要方》济世活人。世人都深为孙思邈的高尚品德和为人处事的精神所感动。

Legend has it that during the reign of Emperor Zhenguan of the Tang Dynasty, Li Shimin's empress had been pregnant for more than ten months and could not give birth and was bedridden. Although treated by many doctors, her condition was never improved. Emperor Taizong sent his envoys to call Sun Simiao into the imperial palace. In feudal societies, due to the restriction of the etiquette of "no physical contact between men and women", when doctors treated intrauterine women, most of them couldn't get close to the patients. A prescription was made at the dictation of others. Sun Simiao called the prime maid of the empress to ask about her conditions and carefully reviewed the prescriptions of the medical records of the former doctors. On the basis of these facts, he acquired a basic knowledge of the empress's illness. Then he took out a red thread and told the maids to tie one end to the empress's wrist with the other end held in his hand and began to feel the "pulse" outside the room. After Sun Simiao finished the diagnosis, he informed Taizong about the etiology and asked the empress to hold the bamboo curtain with her left hand. Sun Simiao saw the acupoint and pricked a needle fiercely. The empress trembled with pain. Soon there came the sound of the baby's cry. The empress gave birth to her son, and she too came to life! Emperor Taizong exulted and invited Sun Simiao to work as an official in the court. But he was determined to cure diseases for the masses and politely declined the position offered by Taizong. Later, he wrote *The Valuable Prescriptions* to save people. People are deeply impressed by Sun Simiao's noble morality and attitudes of doing things.

## 孙思邈——药王医龙的传说

Sun Simiao — The Legend of Treating A Dragon

一日，孙思邈出门，碰见一位穿白衣的少年，跟着许多随从和马匹，迎上前来拜谢孙思邈，说道："小弟承蒙道长相救，父母想见见您。"孙思邈救得人多，听到此话也不当回事。那少年再次恳切邀请，思邈只好上了他准备好的马，和他并驾齐行。那马如飞，一会儿到了一处庄园，望去俨然是王侯府第。少年请孙思邈入内，主人高高兴兴地上来迎接，嘴里谢道："前不久，小儿外出，被人伤害，全靠您保全性命，我们感激先生再生之恩。"孙思邈这才想起来，前不久救活了一条小青蛇，心中十分诧异，问明身边的人才知主人是泾阳龙王！龙王问孙思邈想要什么谢礼，孙思邈回答说："本人只喜好修道，眼中虽看到各种物事，心中却没有什么欲求。"于是龙王命儿子取来秘藏在龙宫的药方三十篇，说："您是真正的有道之士，拿着它们可以济世救人。"于是送孙思邈回到所居的山上。孙思邈对自己遇到的事十分惊异，试着用那三十篇医方治病，效果都很神妙。后来，他编写《千金方》三十卷，将龙宫秘方编入书中。

One day, Sun Simiao met a young man dressed in white who came forward with many followers and horses to bow to Sun Simiao. He said, "My little brother has been saved by you. My parents would like to thank you personally." Sun Simiao had saved many people. Hearing this, he did not take it seriously. The young man asked him earnestly again, so Sun Simiao mounted the horse prepared for him and rode along with the young man. The horse galloped fast and took him to a manor which looked like a royal palace. When the young man invited Sun Simiao inside, the host welcomed him cheerfully and hurriedly thanked, "Not long ago, my child was accidentally hurt. It was lucky of him to have you to save his life. We are grateful for your kindness." Sun Simiao then remembered that he had saved a small green snake. He was very surprised, so he asked the people around him and learned that the host was the Dragon King of Jingyang! The Dragon King asked Sun Simiao what he would want in return. Sun Simiao replied, "Though I have rich life experiences, but I have no desire in me except for practicing medicine." The Dragon King then ordered his son to fetch thirty pieces of prescriptions which were hidden in the dragon palace and sent them to Sun Simiao, saying, "With these you can help people and save them." So the Dragon King sent Sun Simiao back to the mountains where he lived. Sun Simiao was very amazed at what he had encountered. He tried to treat diseases with the thirty prescriptions and they were all very effective. Later, he compiled *The Valuable Prescriptions* in thirty volumes, which included the recipes of the Dragon Palace in the book.

## 第九节 李时珍
### Li Shizhen

李时珍（1518－1593年），湖北蕲春县蕲州镇人，明代著名医药学家。李时珍出生在一个世世代代以行医为业的家族，祖父是一位远近闻名的医生，父亲李言闻对本草学颇有研究。为了了解药性，他的父亲经常到深山老林中搜集药材，这些对幼年的李时珍产生了深远的影响。在父亲的精心指导下，李时珍很快就随着父亲一起出诊了。在多年的医学实践中，李时珍发现古代的本草书籍中有不少的错误，这些错误很可能误人性命。于是他下决心要编撰一部新的本草学书籍。李时珍先后到武当山、庐山、茅山、牛首山及安徽、河南、河北等地收集药物标本和处方，并拜渔人、樵夫、农民、车夫、药工、捕蛇者为师，参考了历代医药方面的书籍约925种，记录了千万字的札记，弄清了许多疑难问题。历经了27个寒暑，三次修改书稿，李时珍于明万历十八年（1590年），在其父亲、儿子及弟子的帮助下，完成了192万字的巨著《本草纲目》。李时珍对脉学、奇经八脉也有研究，另著有《奇经八脉考》等书。

Li Shizhen (1518 A.D. － 1593 A.D.) was a native of Qizhou Town, Qichun County, Hubei Province, a famous practitioner and pharmacist in the Ming Dynasty. Li Shizhen was born in a family that had practiced medicine for generations. His grandfather was a well-known doctor, while Li Yanwen, his father, was an expert in herbology. In order to understand medicinal properties, his father often went deep into the mountains and forests to collect medicinal herbs. His father's deeds had influenced him since his childhood. Under the careful guidance of his father, Li Shizhen treated patients soon with his father. In medical practice, Li Shizhen found that there were many mistakes in ancient herbal books, which might damage the lives of patients. So he made up his mind to compile a new herbology book. Li Shizhen went to Wudang Mountain, Lu Mountain, Mao Mountain, Niushou Mountain as well as Anhui, Henan, Hebei and other places to collect drug specimens and prescriptions. He also asked fishermen, woodcutters, farmers, coachmen, pharmacists, and snake catchers to be his teachers. 925 books on medicine and other aspects of history had been referred to. With archaeological evidence, he took notes of tens of millions of words and clarified many difficult problems. After 27 years, he completed the 1.92-million-word masterpiece with the help of his father, son and disciples in the eighteenth year of the reign of Emperor Wanli in the Ming Dynasty (1590 A.D.). In addition, he also studied the eight extraordinary vessels with his book *On Eight Extraordinary Vessels* as the evidence.

## 《本草纲目》

*Compendium of Materia Medica*

　　《本草纲目》是李时珍同其父其子及弟子，经过27年的长期努力，共同编写，次子建元为书绘图，以李时珍为主的一本集体著作。初稿于明神宗万历六年（1578年）完成。又经过10年三次修改，前后共耗时40年。《本草纲目》共52卷，约190万字。全书收载各家本草药物1518种，在此基础上增收374种，共1892种，其中植物药1195种。此书共编辑了古代药学家的民间单方11096个。这部伟大的著作，吸收了历代本草著作的精华，尽可能地纠正了以前的错误，补充了不足，并有很多重要发现和突破。《本草纲目》是到16世纪为止中国最系统、最完整、最科学的一部医药学著作。李时珍在植物学方面所创造的人为分类方法，是把实用与形态等相似的植物进行归类，这不仅提示了植物之间的亲缘关系，而且还规范了许多植物的命名方法。除本草学的内容以外，还涉及有关动物、天文、地理、化学等方面的知识，英国的博物学家达尔文称《本草纲目》为古代中国的百科全书。

*Compendium of Materia Medica* is a collective work mainly written by Li Shizhen together with his father, son and disciples after 27 years of long-term efforts. His second son Jianyuan drew pictures for the book. The first draft was completed in 1578, the sixth year of the Reign of Emperor Mingshen. After that, it was revised three times in 10 years with a total of 40 years of compilation. *Compendium of Materia Medica* has 52 volumes with about 1.9 million words. In this book, 1,518 kinds of drugs are collected from various herbs, and 374 kinds of drugs are added on the basis of predecessors, totaling 1,892 kinds, including 1,195 kinds of plants. A total of 11,096 items of ancient pharmacists and folk magical prescriptions are compiled. This great work absorbs the essence of all the works of herbology, corrects the mistakes of the past as much as possible, supplements the shortcomings, and makes many important discoveries and breakthroughs. It had been the most systematic, complete and scientific work of medicine by the 16th century in China. The artificial classification method created by Li Shizhen in botany is used to classify a kind of plant into various types according to its practicality and morphology, which not only indicates the kinship of plants, but also standardizes the naming methods of many plants. Apart from the contents of herbology, this book also involves the knowledge of animals, astronomy, geography, chemistry and other aspects, so the British naturalist Charles Darwin called *Compendium of Materia Medica* "the encyclopedia of ancient China".

# 成语故事
## Idioms

## 第一节　讳疾忌医
### Hide One's Sickness for Fear of Treatment

　　《史记·扁鹊仓公列传》记载了扁鹊诊病的一个故事。有一次扁鹊路过齐国，受到齐桓公的接待。扁鹊发现齐桓公面带病色，便劝齐桓公及时治疗，齐桓公不听。扁鹊只好告辞回去了。过了五天，扁鹊拜见齐桓公时说："您现在病位在血脉，不治的话病情会加重。"齐桓公还是没把扁鹊的话当回事。又过了五天左右，扁鹊来拜见齐桓公，这次扁鹊义正词严地对齐桓公讲："您现在病位已深入到肠胃，不治的话就很危险了。"这次齐桓公干脆对扁鹊不理睬了。又过了几天，扁鹊第四次遇到了齐桓公，这次扁鹊转身就走了。齐桓公便好奇地差使下人去问扁鹊。扁鹊说："疾病在腠理，用敷熨的方法可以治疗；疾病在血脉，用针灸可以治疗；疾病在肠胃，用煎药可以治疗；疾病在骨髓，纵然是神仙也没有办法了。现在齐桓公的疾病就深入到了骨髓，已经没救了，我还有什么好说的呢。"五天过后，齐桓公果然重病不起，急忙派人去请扁鹊，这时扁鹊已经逃走了，没过多长时间齐桓公就死了。

这个成语故事告诉我们：有了疾病，应该积极治疗，若讳疾忌医，到头来只会害了自己。

There is a story about Bian Que's diagnosis in *Biography of Bian Que and Cang Gong in the Records of the Historian*. It is about Bian Que who passed by the State of Qi and was welcomed by Duke Huan. When Bian Que found that Duke Huan was looking sickly, he advised him to get prompt treatment, but he did not listen. Bian Que had to leave and go back home. Five days later, Bian Que paid a visit to Duke Huan again. He said, "You are now sick in your blood and vessels. If you don't cure it, your illness will get worse." Duke Huan did not take Bian Que's words seriously. Another five days later, Bian Que came to see Duke Huan. This time, Bian Que said to him in an upright and sincere way, "Now your illness has gone deep into your zangfu organs. It will be very fatal if you don't cure it." Duke Huan simply ignored Bian Que this time. A few days later, Bian Que met Duke Huan for the fourth time. This time Bian Que turned around and left. Duke Huan of Qi then sent his men to ask Bian Que curiously. Bian Que said: "When diseases are in skin, applying plasters can cure you. When diseases are in the blood and vessels, acupuncture and moxibustion are used to treat you. When diseases are in the stomach and intestines, medications can be used. When the disease is in the bone and marrow, even the divine doctors could

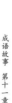

成语故事 第十一章

not save your life. Now your disease has been deep into the bone and marrow, so there is no room to save it. What can I say?" Five days later, Duke Huan was seriously ill, so he sent for Bian Que. By this time Bian Que had already fled. This idiom tells us: if you have a disease, you should treat it positively and actively. If you deny treating it, you will only do harm to yourself in the end.

## 第二节　起死回生
### Bring the Dead Back to Life

　　《史记·扁鹊仓公列传》记载了扁鹊使虢太子"起死回生"的故事。扁鹊是战国时的名医。有一天他经过虢国，听说虢国太子猝死，便来到宫门前，向侍从打听原委。了解了太子的病症，又知其断气不到半天，还未入殓，就跟侍从保证自己可以救回太子。侍从不相信，但听了扁鹊治病的方法，敬佩不已，立刻禀报虢君。虢君赶紧请扁鹊进宫。扁鹊对虢君说："依我看，太子这是尸厥，因体内气血不通而昏死过去，实际上并没有真的死亡，还有机会救回。"于是命令弟子准备好医疗用具，针灸太子的一些穴位。不一会儿，太子就醒过来了。扁鹊再叫弟子用药热敷他的腋下，并将太子扶起坐着，调理身体的阴阳之气。之后再连续服药二十天，太子就完全康复了。经历这件事情，所有人都说扁鹊能让死人复生，但扁鹊却说："不是我能让死人复生，是这人还有机会存活，我才能把他救回而已。"这便是"起死回生"的由来，用来比喻医术高明，也用于比喻将毫无希望的情势扭转过来。

　　In *Biography of Bian Que and Cang Gong in the Records of the Historian,* Sima Qian recorded the story of Bian Que's bringing the dying prince of Guo State back to life. Bian Que was a famous doctor in the Warring States Period. One day when he passed through the State of Guo, he heard that the prince had died suddenly, so he went to the palace gate and asked the prince's attendants about the fact. He learnt that the prince had been dead for no more than half a day and had not yet been buried. From the symptoms described by the attendants, he was confident to promise that he could rescue him. They did not believe it, but after hearing Bian Que's therapeutic method, astounded, they immediately reported to the King of Guo State who invited Bian Que to the palace. Bian Que said, "From my point of view, the prince is suffering from necropia. In fact, he has not really died. There's still a chance to get it back." Then he ordered the disciples to prepare some medical equipment and manipulate the prince's points by acupuncture. After a while, the prince woke up. Bian Que then asked the disciple to warm his armpits with medications alternately, and helped the prince to sit up and recuperate his yin and yang. After taking drugs for another 20 days, the prince recovered completely. Since then, everyone said Bian Que could bring a dead man back to life, but Bian Que said, "I can not make it, but that I can save the dead man while he still has a chance to live." From here comes the idiom "bring the dead back to life", which is used to describe a person of high skills in medicine. It is also used figuratively when a hopeless situation can be turned around.

## 第三节　肝胆相照
## Sworn Brothers

　　"肝胆相照"的成语故事最早记录于《史记·淮阴侯列传》中。韩信因其杰出的军事才华和雄才大略被汉王刘邦重用。对于当时纷乱的天下局势，韩信起着重要的作用，楚、汉无论哪一方得到他诚心的辅佐，都有可以夺得天下。有一个叫蒯（kuǎi）通的谋士，劝韩信背叛汉王刘邦，自立为王，与汉王、楚王三分天下，形成鼎立之势。蒯通说："我愿意披肝沥胆，敬献愚计，只恐怕您不采纳啊。"蒯通以肝和胆的密切关系做比喻，来向韩信表示自己的衷心与诚恳。中医理论阐释，肝胆生理功能关系极为密切，互为表里。人体的情志活动中，肝主疏泄，肝藏血，其气升发，喜条达而恶抑郁。中医认为肝负责思索谋虑，胆负责决断，二者相互配合，使人能做出决定而不至于怯懦。在经络循行中，足少阳胆经和足厥阴肝经相连，相互络属。肝胆在解剖结构、生理功能、经络循行上都有着密切的关系。肝胆相照，本意是肝与胆相互照应，常用来比喻可以相互坦诚交往与共事。

　　The story of this idiom was first recorded in *Marquis Huaiyin Biographies of Historical Records*. Han Xin, was entrusted with an important post by Liu Bang, the King of Han, because of his outstanding military talent. Han Xin played an important role in the turbulent world at that time. Either Chu or Han got his sincere assistance, they would certainly win the world. A counsellor named Kuai Tong tried to persuade Han Xin to rebel against the King of Han and make himself the king by splitting himself with both Han and Chu. Kuai said, "I want to exhaust myself to give all my advice, but I fear you will not accept it." He expressed his sincerity to Han Xin with a figure of speech as close relationship between the liver and gallbladder. TCM theory explains that the physiological function of the liver and gallbladder is closely related to each other. In the human body's emotional activities, the liver dominates free flow with its qi likely to rise and disperse. It dislikes stagnation and depression. The gallbladder is responsible for thought and courage for decision. If the two work together so that one can make decisions without cowardice. As for the meridian, the gallbladder meridian of the foot shaoyang and the liver meridian of the foot jueyin are closely connected. The liver and the gallbladder have a close relationship in anatomical structure, physiological function and meridian. The idiom means that the liver and the gallbladder take care of each other. The implication is to be honest with each other and work with each other.

## 第四节　病入膏肓
### The Disease Has Attacked the Vitals

"病入膏肓"出自《左传·成公十年》，意思是病情特别严重，无法医治，也比喻事态严重到不可挽回的地步。春秋时期晋景公得了一场病，请了很多医生都看不好，他就从邻国请了一个叫医缓的大夫。大夫还在来的路上的时候，晋景公做了一个梦。他梦见两个小孩，这两个小孩说："那位医生就要来了，咱俩赶快藏起来吧，不能让那个大夫找到咱们，咱们藏到膏肓那个地方他就找不着我们了。"等医缓来了诊脉后，对景公说："这病不好治了，已入膏肓，吃药不行，针灸也不行，没治了。"后人认为，膏指心尖的油脂，肓指心外膜。膏肓是很危险的地方，药到不了，针不能扎。另一种解释是膏肓指一个穴位，大概在人肩胛骨内侧。在日常养生保健中，可以对膏肓穴进行艾灸。一般采用艾条灸，灸10～15分钟，以皮肤温热微红为宜。历代医家多认为，灸膏肓穴可补益虚损、调养心肺，可放松肩背、缓解肩背疼痛，同时也可以有效地预防心、肺疾病。

The idiom "The Disease has attacked the vitals" is from *Zuo Zhuan · Tenth Year of Duke Cheng*. It means that the disease is so serious that it can't be cured. In the Spring and Autumn Period, the Duke Jing of the State of Jin fell ill. Many doctors could not cure him so he sent for a doctor from a neighboring state called Huan. While the doctor was still on his way, the Duke Jing had a dream in which two little children said: "The doctor is coming. Let's hide quickly. We can't let the doctor find us." When the doctor felt his pulse, he said to the Duke: "This disease is incurable. It is already on the verge of death even with herbs or acupuncture." Later, people know that "gao(膏)" refers to fat at the apex of the heart, "huang (肓)" refers to the pericardium. "Gaohuang" refers to a very important place in human body that herbs and acupuncture couldn't easily work. Another interpretation refers to an acupuncture point below the scapula. In daily health care, moxibustion can be carried out for Gaohuang acupoints. Generally use moxa strips to manipulate the point for 10 to 15 minutes till the skin is warm and reddish. Medical experts in the past dynasties believed that this point had the effect of tonifying deficiency and nourishing the heart and lung. Moxibustion on Gaohuang point can not only relax one's shoulder and back and relieve it of pain, but also can effectively prevent the cardiac and pulmonary diseases.

## 第五节　良药苦口
### A Good Medicine Tastes Bitter

中国有句古话"良药苦口利于病，忠言逆耳利于行"。这句话最早出自《史记·留侯世家》。沛公刘邦进入秦朝的咸阳宫后，被宫中的美色珍玩吸引，忘乎所以，张良入宫直谏，说了这句话。这句话的意思是良药多数是带苦味的，却对治病利；而教人从善的语言多数是不太动听的，但有利于人们改正缺点。这句贤文旨在教育人们要勇于接受批评，正确地对待别人的意见和批评。因为一个人有过错并不可怕，只要能够及时地改正就无大碍，可怕的是不愿意接受别人的批评意见，以至于由小错到大错，由大错到不可救药。苦药虽然很难让人下咽，却有利于自己治病，忠言虽然有点逆耳，但能帮助纠正言行。一个人活在世上，能够得到智者的批评和指导是一件幸事。

There is an old Chinese saying that "good medicine is bitter in the mouth but beneficial to curing the disease; while good advice goes against the ear but helps to act." It originally came from *Marquis Liu Family of Historical Records*. It tells the story that after Liu Bang entered the Xianyang Palace of the Qin Dynasty, he was carried away by the beauty and curios in the palace. Zhang Liang remonstrated with him by saying that "good medicine tastes bitter but is beneficial to curing the disease; while good advice helps to act in spite of its strict criticism." This means that good medicine, mostly bitter, is good for healing; sincere speech is not pleasant to listen, but it helps people to correct their shortcomings. The virtuous words aim at educating people to be brave to accept critics. It is often used to show that one should treat the opinions and criticism of others correctly, for a man's faults are not terrible as long as he corrects it in time. The terrible thing is not to accept criticism so that a small mistake becomes a big one, and a big one becomes impossible to correct. Bitter medicine, though hard to swallow, is good for healing. Unpleasant words, though hurtful, can help us in every deed. It is a blessing for a man to have the criticism and guidance of wise men.

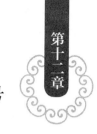

# 象征符号
## Symbols

## 第一节　太极图
### Taiji Diagram

　　太极图是以黑白两个鱼形纹组成的图案，鱼形纹俗称阴阳鱼。太极是中国古代的哲学术语，是指产生万物的本源。太极图有以下含义：（1）图中的"S"线将太极图清晰地分为两个部分，表明任何事物的内部都是有结构的。（2）太极图的两个部分用不同颜色来区别，即阴和阳，以"S"线相隔，表明这两个部分是相互独立、不容混淆的。（3）太极图的两个独立部分各有一个对方的小点，即阳中有阴，阴中有阳，表明同一事物结构中的独立部分与对方有包含关系。（4）太极图是圆形图，表明运动和结构有规则，运动以旋转为基本形式以及运动是流畅圆润的。（5）太极图是对称图，表明一个稳定的结构其内部能量是均衡的。（6）太极图中的阴和阳都有大头和小尾的形状，表明事物运动是有方向性的。还表示阴和阳在旋转中的强弱变化，大头为强，小尾为弱，在大头处有对方的小点，同时与对方的小尾衔接，这显示了太极内部两种能量的变化由小到大，又由大到互变的变易性，呈现出物极必反的状态。

The taiji diagram is a pattern composed of a black and a white fish, commonly known as yin and yang fish. Taiji is an ancient Chinese philosophical term meaning the source from which all things derive. The symbol of taiji has the following meanings: (1) The curved line in the taiji diagram clearly divides it into two parts, indicating that everything has a structure inside. (2) The two parts are distinguished by two colors, symbolizing yin and yang, separated by a curved line and indicating that the two parts are independent from each other and cannot be mixed. (3) Each independent part has a small dot of the other side, that is, there is yin in yang and yang in yin, indicating that the independent part in the structure of the same thing is inclusively related with the other side. (4) The taiji diagram is circular, showing the regular movement and structure. Motion is based on smooth rotation. (5) The taiji diagram is symmetric, which indicates that the internal energy of a stable structure is balanced. (6) The yin and yang blocks both have the shape of a big head and a small tail, indicating that things move in a directional manner. It also indicates that the strength of yin and yang changes in rotation, with the big head being strong and the small tail weak. In the big head, there are dots of the other side, and at the same time, they connect with the tail of the other side, which shows the change of the two forces in taiji from small to large, and from large to mutual change. It presents a reverse state when things go too far.

## 第二节　杏林文化
### Apricot Wood Culture

数千年来，代表祖国传统医学的杏林文化从庐山产生并传承至今。杏林文化的开山鼻祖董奉，与南阳的张仲景、谯郡的华佗齐名，并称为东汉末年"建安三神医"。杏林佳话，不仅成为民间和医界的美谈，也成为历代医家激励自己，努力提高医技，解除病人痛苦的典范，"杏林"也成了中医学界的代名词。医家以位列"杏林中人"为荣，医著以"杏林医案"为藏，医技以"杏林圣手"为赞，医德以"杏林春暖"为誉，医道以"杏林养生"为崇。董奉的杏林园创立于1800多年前的东汉末年。董奉在庐山几十年，追求的是"奉天地顺五行"，在现实中构建"和谐杏林园"，从而达到他修道从医的最高境界——无为而为。"杏林"有着"亲、善、诚、信、中、和"的丰富内涵，其灵魂是"道"与"德"。凡习医药者必推崇"杏林精神"，这正是杏林文化延续至今的生命力，同时也是传统中医药文化精神的开宗。

For thousands of years, the culture of Apricot Wood on behalf of traditional Chinese medicine has existed in Lu Mountain and has been passed down to this day. Dong Feng, the founder of Xinglin Culture, with Zhang Zhongjing of Nanyang and Hua Tuo of Qiao County, was known as one of "The Three Magic Doctors of Jian' an" in the late Eastern Han Dynasty. "Apricot Wood" has not only been a beautiful story among ordinary people and the medical field, but also a guidance for physicians in all dynasties to motivate and urge themselves to strive to improve their medical skills and relieve patients' sufferings. It has also become a synonym of the medical profession. Its cultural connotation in some Chinese idioms as "杏林中人" "杏林医案" "杏林圣手" "杏林春暖" "杏林养生" shows doctors' sense of honor, emphasis on ancient medical classics, high-leveled medical skills, morality and ways of health care. Dong Feng's Xinglin garden was founded more than 1,800 years ago in the late Eastern Han Dynasty. He spent several decades on Lu Mountain, pursuing to "respect nature and follow the law of the five elements" and building "a harmonious Apricot Wood garden" in real life so as to reach the highest state of practicing medicine － Inaction. Xinglin embodies a kind of moral standard, which contains the connotation of "amity, kindness, sincerity, faith, mediumness and harmony" and its essence is "Daoism" and "morality". Those who practice medicine will praise the "spirit of the Apricot Wood", which is exactly where the vitality of Xinglin culture continues to this day, and it is also the spiritual essence of traditional Chinese medicine.

## 第三节　龟
### Turtles

　　龟是地球上最古老的动物之一。龟的长寿，与鹤齐名，在古人的心目中龟是长寿的象征。将龟和鼎一样视为国家重器，合称为"龟鼎"。古人还把龟、龙、凤凰和麒麟作为吉祥的动物。早在夏代，人们就将龟视为灵物。有资料表明，夏代已用龟甲占卜了，但从二里头遗址发现的龟甲一般未经整治，有灼无钻。到殷商时期，人们则把龟腹甲整治凿孔，以火灼裂，视其裂纹，占卜吉凶，谓之龟卜。然后，在龟甲上契刻卜辞和少量记事文字，这种文字就是甲骨文。在甲骨文中有不少卜辞提及龟。汉代也视龟为灵物，以龟之形制作兵符用以调兵遣将，并在各级官印上雕以龟饰。唐代女皇武则天认为龟是介虫之长，灵而有寿，就将原来五品以上官员所佩的鱼形袋一律改为龟形，并按不同级别分为金龟袋、银龟袋、铜龟袋三等。到了宋代，苏东坡、陆游等文人学子的帽子上也配上了龟甲。龟是长寿的象征，得天地之阴气尤厚。人们为了延年益寿，龟为药食两用之品，其补益、抗衰老等作用也逐步载入历代医籍。

　　Turtles are among the oldest animals on earth. They are as famous as cranes for their longevity and of longevity symbol in the eyes of the ancients. Turtles and "鼎 dǐng" were regarded as the objects of national importance, known as the "turtle ding". The ancient also regarded turtles, dragons, phoenixes and qilin as the auspicious animals. As early as the Xia Dynasty, people took turtles as the spiritual objects. The data showed that the tortoise shells had been used for divination in the Xia Dynasty, but the tortoise shells found in Erlitou site were generally unprocessed and had been burned with no drill marks. In the Shang Dynasty, people cut holes in their belly bones, split them with fire and divined good or evil by observing their cracks. That is called the turtle divination. Then they carved inscriptions on the tortoise shells and a small amount of writing, which were oracle-bone inscriptions. There are many inscriptions on oracle bones that refer to turtles. The Han Dynasty also regarded turtles as spiritual objects, made a military symbol in the shape of turtles to mobilize troops and engraved on the seals of officials at all levels with turtles as decorations. Empress Wu Zetian of the Tang Dynasty considered turtles to be the leaders of all carapace animals so that they could be immortal and live a long life. So she changed all the fish-shaped bags worn by the officials above the fifth grade to turtle-shaped ones, which were identified by three kinds of material: gold, silver and copper corresponding to different grades. In the Song Dynasty, the hats of scholars such as Su Dongpo and Lu You were decorated with tortoises. A turtle is a symbol of longevity because of its getting much yin qi in nature. In order to prolong people's life, turtles are also used as medicine and food, and their tonic and anti-aging effects have also been gradually recorded in the medical classics of dynasties.

象征符号 第十二章

# 第四节　寿星公
## The Longevity God

中国有"福""禄""寿"三星。寿星公，又称南极仙翁，一直被中国人视作吉祥、长寿的象征。寿星公为白须老翁，手持桃木杖，常以鹿、鹤、仙桃等来衬托。关于寿星公的大脑门儿，有多种猜测，有人认为大脑门儿是返老还童现象，老人和小孩有诸多体貌特征上的相似。比如初生婴儿头发稀少，老年人也是一样。而头发少自然额头就显得很大。另一种说法是：由于道教养生观念的融入，寿星公最突出的特征就是他硕大无比的脑门儿。山西永乐宫壁画中的寿星公，可能是存世最古老的寿星形象。在永乐宫上千位神仙中，我们一眼就能认出他，就是因为他独特的大脑门儿。寿星公的大脑门儿，也与古代养生术所营造的长寿意象紧密相关。比如丹顶鹤的头部高高隆起，再如寿桃是王母娘娘蟠桃会上特供的长寿仙果。传说是蟠桃树三千年一开花，三千年一结果，食用蟠桃后可长生不老。或许就是因为这些长寿意象融合叠加，最终造就了寿星公的大脑门儿。

In mythology, China has three gods: "福fu", "禄lu" and "寿shou" among which the longevity god is also known as the Antarctic fairy on behalf of the elderly. He has been also regarded as a symbol of good luck. The longevity god is an old man with white beard, usually deer, cranes and peaches beside him, holding a peach stick. There are many speculations as to the origin of his large forehead. It has been suggested that the large forehead is the result of a phenomenon known as rejuvenation with older people and young children sharing many physical and facial features. For example, newborns have thinning hair, and so do older adults. With less hair, he obviously has a large forehead. Another saying of it is that the most prominent feature of the longevity god is his huge forehead due to the integration of Taoist health concepts. The longevity figure in the mural of Yongle Palace in Shanxi is probably the oldest one in existence. Among the thousands of immortals in Yongle Palace, we can recognize him immediately because of his super forehead. The huge forehead of the longevity god is also closely related to the image of longevity created by ancient health preservation techniques. For example, the forehead of the red-crowned crane is high raised, and the longevity peach is the immortal fruit specially offered by the Queen Mother of the West. Legend has it that the immortal peach trees bloom every 3,000 years and harvest in another 3000 years. People who eat one of them would become immortal. Perhaps it is the combination of these longevity images that ultimately results in the longevity god's large forehead.

## 第五节　寿桃

**A Peach for Longevity**

中国神话中，寿桃是令人延年益寿的桃子。寿桃也指祝寿所用的桃，一般用面粉做成，也有用鲜桃的。为什么桃子在贺寿之时有重要的地位呢？这大概同古代人民对桃树的信仰及西王母的神话传说有关系。神话中，西王母娘娘做寿，设蟠桃会款待群仙，所以民间习俗就用桃来做庆寿的物品。现在人们也有用玉石、红木来雕成寿桃的样子。每当老年人过生日时，做儿女的都会送寿桃给老人，以祝老人健康、长寿、幸福。而旧时人们认为，老人吃了寿桃会变年轻进而长寿。现代研究表明，桃味道甜、鲜，纤维素含量高，含有维生素E，具有抗氧化、抗衰老的作用，果糖又有滋补强身的作用，特别是纤维素对老人的常见病如动脉硬化、便秘都有好处。民间早有"桃养人，杏伤人"和"宁吃鲜桃一口，不吃烂杏一筐"的谚语。

A peach for longevity is a peach in Chinese mythology that can prolong one's life. Longevity peach also refers to the peach served for birthday, usually made of flour or fresh peach. Why do peaches play such an important role in celebrating longevity? This may have something to do with the ancient people's belief in peach trees and the myth and legend of the Queen Mother of the West. In mythology, the Queen Mother of the West treated the fairies with peaches on her birthday, so peaches were commonly used as birthday objects. Now people also make longevity peaches with materials like jade or mahogany. Whenever an old man celebrates his birthday, the children will send longevity peaches to the old man to express the wish of health, longevity and happiness. In the old days, it was believed that old people who ate longevity peaches would grow younger and live longer. Modern research shows that peaches are sweet, fresh and rich in cellulose. They contain vitamin E which is antioxidant and anti-aging. Fructose plays the role of nourishing and strengthening the body and especially cellulose is beneficial to the prevention of common diseases such as arteriosclerosis and constipation for the elderly. There has long been folk proverbs "a peach nourishes one's body" and "would rather eat a mouthful of fresh peach than a basket of rotten apricots".

第
十
三
章

# 历史痕迹
## Traces of History

## 第一节　中国古代医学分科
### Subspecialty of Ancient Chinese Medicine

　　早在周代（公元前1046年 — 公元前256年），我国就已经出现了医学分科。《周礼》一书全面地反映了西周时期的社会情况，其中记载周朝医学分为四科，即食、疾、疡、兽，意思是食医、疾医、疡医、兽医，相当于现代的营养师、内科医生、外科医生和兽医。随着朝代的更替，医学分科不断细化。唐代由政府设立的太医署，是当时医疗行政和医学教育的最高机构，就有医科、针科、按摩科、咒禁科。针对临床医疗又分为体疗（内科）、少小（儿科）、疮肿（外科）、耳目口齿（五官口腔科）、角法（外治法）。宋代政府设立了翰林医官院，设有九科，即大方脉（内科）、风科、小方脉（小儿科）、疮肿兼折疡、眼科、产科、口齿兼咽喉科、针灸科、金镞兼书禁科。元代时期，由于骑术盛行和战争频繁，骨折外伤病人明显增多，正骨科单独成科。此时的医学分为十三科，即大方脉、杂医科、小方脉科、风科、产科、眼科、口齿科、咽喉科、正骨科、金疮肿科、针灸科、祝由科、禁科。明清两代基本沿袭元代分科，无太大改变。

As early as the Zhou Dynasty from 1046 B.C. to 256 B.C., medical branches appeared in China. *The Rites of Zhou* comprehensively reflected the social situation of the Western Zhou Dynasty. Medicine in the Zhou Dynasty was divided into four branches, namely, diet, diseases, sores, animals, which meant departments dealing with diet therapy, internal illnesses, surgical problems and sickness in animals. They are the modern equivalents of nutritionists, physicians, surgeons and veterinarians respectively. With the change of dynasties, medical branches developed continuously and respectively. The Imperial Hospital established by the government in the Tang Dynasty represented the highest institution of medical administration and medical education at that time including departments of medicine, acupuncture, massage and incantation. Clinical treatment was divided into body therapy (internal medicine), kids (pediatrics), sores and swelling (surgery), eyes and ears (five senses and stomatology department), rectification method (external treatment). The government of the Song Dynasty established the Hanlin Medical Academy including nine departments: internal medicine, wind, pediatrics, sores and acne, ophthalmology, obstetrics, oral and larynx, acupuncture, zhuyou. In the Yuan Dynasty, due to the prevalence of riding and frequent wars, the number of fracture injuries increased significantly and orthopedics became a separate department.

At this time, medicine was divided into 13 departments including internal medicine, miscellaneous medicine, pediatrics, wind, obstetrics, ophthalmology, stomatology, laryngology, orthopedics, wounds and sores, acupuncture and moxibustion, zhuyou and incantation. The Ming and Qing Dynasties followed the practice of the Yuan Dynasty and did not make many changes.

## 第二节 古代女子美颜离不开益母草
## Motherwort － The Beauty Treatment of Ancient Women

对于古代人使用的化妆品，人们会想到铅粉，但铅粉含有轻微的铅毒，长期使用对人体有害，会让肤色发黑，于是古人便在自然界中寻找各种成本低廉，同时又具有营养或治疗功效的原料。益母草灰正是在这种背景下被开发出来的一种营养妆粉，宋人还为之起了一个特别诗意的名字——"玉女粉"。现代药典记载，益母草含有多种微量元素，有抗氧化、防衰老和抗癌功效。益母草是一种生命力极强的野草，在田间野外随处可见，因此，当人们需要的时候，能很容易地找到这种美容原料，也可以大量地采摘收集。商家把多种中草药与益母草相配，制成复杂、高档的美容用品，但普通的家庭主妇、民间少女也能自己动手制作"玉女粉"：采来益母草，烧成灰，再加入米粥中煮一下，然后连粥捏成团，到炭火中煅烧一番，随后取出，待凉后研成细粉，就大功告成了，任何一个平民妇女凭借自家的火炉或烧饭灶都可以轻松制作。

For cosmetics used in ancient times, people tend to think of lead powder. However, lead powder contains slight lead poison, which is harmful to the human body and darkens the skin after a long-term use. Therefore, ancient people looked for all kinds of raw materials in nature that were cheap but had nutritional or therapeutic effects. Such a nutritious makeup powder was just developed out of motherwort. People in the Song Dynasty also gave it a special poetic name — "powder for fairies". Modern pharmacopoeia also records motherwort contains a variety of trace elements with antioxidant, anti-aging and even anti-cancer effects. Motherwort is a hardy weed that grows in fields. As a result, when ancient people needed it, they could easily find this beauty ingredient and collected them in large quantities. Doctors and merchants could combine a variety of Chinese herbs and motherwort to make sophisticated, high-end beauty products while ordinary housewives and folk girls could also pick such weeds and make "powder for fairies" by themselves: gather motherwort and burn them to ashes, add them to the rice porridge and cook it, then make a ball of porridge, calcine it in a charcoal fire, then take it out, let it cool and grind it to a fine powder. Then it was done! Any civilian woman could make it easily with her own stove for cooking.

## 第三节　古代医生的各种称呼
### Address Forms of Doctors in Ancient China

　　古代对于医者的称呼多与官职有关，例如"大夫"，最初就是官名，读作dà fū；读作dài fu时，指医生，始于宋代。"郎中"，起初也是官名，即帝王侍从官的通称。战国时就开始有这种官职了。郎中作为医生的称呼也始于宋代，南方习惯称医生为郎中。"医生"这个词始于唐代。推测是古代太医署"医学生"的简称。古时候，对周游于农村城市，具有一技之长，并以串铃召呼病家的医生，称为走方医或铃医。这些人的医术大多来自师传口授，使用少数草药和简便的医疗方法来治病救人。坐堂医是指在中药店中为患者诊脉看病的中医大夫。相传汉代名医张仲景为长沙太守时，每月的初一和十五坐堂行医，并分文不取。为了纪念张仲景崇高的医德和高超的医术，后来许多中药店都冠以某某堂，并把坐在药铺里诊病的医师称为"坐堂医"，这种称呼沿用至今。御医是古时候专门为皇帝及其宫廷亲属治病的宫廷医师。巫医是比一般巫师更专门于医药的人物。

　　In ancient times, a doctor's name was mostly related to an official position. For example, "大夫" originally an official name, was pronounced as "dà fū". When pronounced as "dài fū", it refers to a doctor, which can date back to the Song Dynasty. "Langzhong", originally was the official name, namely the general name of the imperial chamberlain official. This kind of official position has existed since the Warring States Period. The name of "Langzhong", known as a doctor also began in the Song Dynasty, and it was customary to call a doctor "Langzhong" in the southern area of China. The word "医生" originated in the Tang Dynasty. It was the abbreviation of "medical students" of the ancient Department of Imperial Medicine. In ancient times, those who traveled in the countryside and cities, had a medical skill and appealed to the patient with a bell were known as "走方医" (moving doctors) or "铃医" (bell doctors). Most of their medical knowledge was acquired by dictation from their teachers, who used a few herbs and simple remedies for saving people. "坐堂医" is a TCM doctor who took a patient's pulse in a TCM pharmacy. It is said that Zhang Zhongjing, a famous doctor in the Han Dynasty and the Changsha satrap usually sat in the government office treating patients in his sparetime without taking any medical charge on the first and fifteenth of every lunar month. In order to commemorate Zhang Zhongjing's lofty medical ethics and superb medical skills, many Chinese pharmacies later got their names containing the Chinese character "堂tang" and referred to the doctors who sat in the pharmacy as "坐堂医". The term is still used today. "御医" was a court physician who treated the emperor and his relatives in ancient times. A witch doctor was a person more specialized in medicine than an average sorcerer.

# 第四节　古代的医院类型
## Types of Ancient Hospitals

　　我国古代的医院有多种多样的形式。春秋初期管仲创建了养病的场所，收容聋哑人、盲人、跛足者、疯人和残疾人。这是在中国出现最早的有记载的医院萌芽。此后，隋、唐、宋、元、明、清各朝代都有公立或私立的养病场所。我国很早就认识到疾病的传染性并采取了相应的隔离措施，这种类似的"时疫医院"最早出现于西汉。从隋唐时代，我国开始设置麻风病院，叫作"疠人坊"。从两晋、南北朝到隋唐时代，佛教鼎盛，印度医学也随佛教转入我国。不少佛教徒以医传教，有的兼做医生，到附近山上采药。病人也常去求诊，寺院也渐渐开始收住病人。古代的医药成果一直被统治阶级占有，因而宫廷医学被奉为正统医学。我国自秦汉以来的历代王朝，都设有为皇室贵族服务的医疗组织，如太医署、太医院、御药院等，这里集中着一批医生，随时奉诏为皇室贵族和封建官僚诊治疾病。另外，古代战争频繁，造成了大批伤病员。东汉时有类似军医院的机构，叫"庵庐"。元代以后，这种机构进一步健全，改名为"安乐堂"。

Hospitals in ancient China had many forms. At the beginning of the Spring and Autumn Period, Guan Zhong set up a place of convalescence for the deaf, the blind, the lame, the mad and the disabled. This is one of the earliest hospitals in China. Thereafter, the Sui, Tang, Song, Yuan, Ming and Qing dynasties all had public or private places for the sick to recuperate. China has long recognized the infectivity of some diseases and their isolation measures. This kind of similar "epidemic hospital" first appeared in the Western Han Dynasty. Since the Sui and Tang Dynasties, our country has started to set up leprosy hospitals. From the Jin, Northern and Southern Dynasties to the Sui and Tang dynasties, Buddhism reached its peak, and Indian medicine was transferred to China along with Buddhism. Many Buddhists preached combined with medicine. They even went to the nearby mountains to collect herbs. So patients often went to seek treatment in the temple, which also gradually admitted patients. The medical resources were always possessed by the ruling class, so court medicine was regarded as orthodox medicine. Since the Qin and Han dynasties, there were medical organizations for the royal family, such as the Imperial Medical Bureau and imperial pharmacies. Here gathered a group of doctors, who always diagnosed and treated diseases for the royal family and feudal officials. In addition, the frequent wars in ancient times caused a large number of casualties. In the Eastern Han Dynasty, there were institutions similar to military hospitals, called "Anlu". After the Yuan Dynasty, this kind of organization was further improved and renamed as "Anle Hall".

# 第五节　中国针灸对外传播之路
## Overseas Spread of Acupuncture

　　纵观针灸对外传播的历史，大致可以划分为三个阶段。第一阶段：6世纪左右至15世纪末，约1000年。针灸在朝鲜半岛、日本、越南、印度尼西亚等地区传播。针灸向西域的传播则很有限。自汉代开始，古人就开辟了沟通中亚、西亚、南亚直至地中海东岸的陆路和海上通道，被后人称为"丝绸之路"。第二阶段：16世纪初至1970年，约500年。早期主要传播到荷兰、法国、英国、德国、意大利等欧洲国家，并在19世纪初通过欧洲传播到美国、澳大利亚和俄罗斯等国。后期从1963年开始，中国政府派遣的援非医疗队将针灸传播到很多非洲国家。第三阶段：1971年至今，仅仅50年。这几十年时间里，针灸就已经传播到140多个国家和地区，约占全世界国家和地区总数的三分之二。在现代针灸对外传播历史上，1971年是个分水岭。在此之前，针灸只在少数国家流传，而在此之后则形成一股世界性的"针灸热"，势不可挡，持续至今。

　　The history of acupuncture spread overseas can be roughly divided into three stages. The first period is from about the 6th century to the end of the 15th century, covering about 1,000 years. During this period, acupuncture was spread in the Korean Peninsula, Japan, Vietnam, Indonesia and other regions. The spread to the western regions was limited then. Since the Han Dynasty, land and sea routes have been opened to connect, Central Asia, West Asia and South Asia to the eastern coast of the Mediterranean Sea, which later became known as the Silk Road. The second period is from the early 16th century to 1970, covering about 500 years. It was mainly spread to the Netherlands, France, Britain, Germany, Italy and other European countries in the early 19th century and later to the United States, Australia, Russia and other countries through Europe. Later, beginning in 1963, the Chinese government sent medical teams to provide acupuncture service for people in many African countries. The third period from 1971 to now is only more than 50 years. Over the past few decades, acupuncture has spread to more than 140 countries and regions, accounting for about two-thirds of the world's total. In the history of modern acupuncture, 1971 was a watershed year. Before that, acupuncture was only spread in a few countries, but after that, there formed a worldwide "acupuncture craze", which is unstoppable and continues to this day.

## 第六节 《黄帝内经》
### *Huangdi Neijing*

《黄帝内经》分《灵枢》和《素问》两部分，是古代医家托黄帝之名而作，一般认为成书于春秋战国时期。以黄帝、岐伯、雷公问答的形式阐述病因病机，此著作主张不治已病，而治未病，同时主张养生、摄生、益寿、延年。它是中国传统医学四大经典著作之一，是我国医学宝库中现存成书最早的一部医学典籍。内容包括生理学、病理学、诊断学、治疗原则和药物学，在理论上建立了中医学上的"阴阳五行学说""脉象学说""藏象学说"等。有学者形象地称《黄帝内经》是"以生命为中心的百科全书"。在商周时期，医学仍以鬼神观念占居统治地位，不仅病因要寻求鬼神作用的因素，治疗也多用巫术。到了《黄帝内经》形成的时期，这种认识逐渐发生了转变，围绕着疾病诊疗是否鬼神因素在理论和实践上展开了激烈的争论。民间医生扁鹊及《内经》的作者们在这场影响深远的斗争中，鲜明地反对鬼神说。

*Huangdi Neijing (Inner Canon of Huangdi)* is divided into two parts: *Plain Questions* and *Miraculous Pivot*. It is generally believed that it was composed in the Spring and Autumn Period and Warring States Period in the name of Huangdi. While explaining the etiology and pathogenesis in the form of questions and answers from Huangdi, Qibo and Lei Gong, it focuses on more of the preventive treatment than a disease you have already had and at the same time advocates keeping healthy and prolonging life. It is one of the four classical works of traditional Chinese medicine and the earliest medical book in China. It is a medical masterpiece on human physiology, pathology, diagnostics, therapeutic principles and pharmacology. It establishes the theories of yin and yang and five elements, the pulse theory and the theory of visceral manifestation. Some scholars vividly consider *Huangdi Neijing* "the life-centered encyclopedia". In the Period of the Shang and Zhou dynasties, the concept of ghosts and spirits was still in the dominant position. In the period of the formation of *Huangdi Neijing*, this kind of understanding was gradually changed, and there was a fierce debate on the theory and practice about whether the diagnosis and treatment of diseases were associated with ghosts. Bian Que, a folk doctor, and the authors of *Neijing* were opposed to the doctrine of ghosts in this far-reaching struggle.

## 第七节　人痘接种术
**Vaccine for Smallpox**

天花是一种烈性传染病，病人死亡率非常高。长期以来，人类一直没有有效的防治方法。我国古代人民在"以毒攻毒"的思想指导下，于明代发明了人痘接种法。人痘接种使千千万万的人们，免除了天花的威胁和侵害。它的发明，同活字印刷、造纸术、火药、指南针四大发明一样，是中国人民对人类的伟大贡献。清康熙二十七年（1688年），俄国医生来到北京学习人痘接种法。18世纪中叶，人痘接种法传遍欧亚大陆。我国的人痘接种术对英国医生琴纳发明牛痘接种术启发很大。他八岁时曾接种过人痘，接种后感觉很不舒服，便产生了改良种痘方法的念头。有一次，他发现牛也会生天花，并可以传染给人，但出痘很少，症状很轻，几乎没有什么痛苦，人也同样获得对天花的免疫力。为此他进行了八年的试验，终于在1796年，他获得了成功。从此牛痘接种术逐渐取代了人痘接种法。1805年牛痘接种术又传入我国。因为牛痘接种术比人痘接种法更加安全，我国也逐渐用种牛痘取替了种人痘，由此改进了种痘技术。

Smallpox was a virulent infectious disease with a very high mortality rate in the past. For a long time, there had been no effective preventive method. Under the guidance of "like cures like", the ancient Chinese people invented the method of inoculation with human pox in the Ming Dynasty. Smallpox inoculation freed millions of people from the threat of smallpox. Its invention, like the four great inventions of movable type printing, papermaking, gunpowder and compass, is the great contribution of the Chinese people to mankind. In the twenty-seventh year of Kangxi's reign in 1688, Russian doctors came to Beijing to learn how to inoculate with human pox. In the mid-18th century, vaccinations spread across Eurasia. This type of vaccination inspired the invention of vaccinia by the English doctor Jenner. He was vaccinated against smallpox when he was eight years old. He felt very uncomfortable after the inoculation and had the idea to reform the vaccination method. On one occasion, he discovered that cows had smallpox too, and that it could be transmitted to humans, but with few outbreaks, mild symptoms and little pain and that humans had also acquired immunity to smallpox. He experimented for eight years, and finally, in 1796, he achieved success. Since then vaccinia inoculation gradually replaced artificial inoculation. Vaccination was introduced into China in 1805. Because vaccinia was safer than human pox, our country gradually replaced it with vaccinia and improved vaccination technology.

## 第八节　少林伤科
### Shaolin Orthopedics and Traumatology

提到少林，大家印象非常深刻的就是少林功夫，其历史底蕴非常深厚，是我国传统武术的重要组成部分，自古就有"天下武功出少林"的说法。少林文化所包含的可不仅仅是武术，在其理念体系中，少林伤科同样是重要的医学分支。在数千年的演化过程中，已经成为中华骨伤科中最有影响力的一个流派，如果说天下武功出自少林，那么天下伤科亦出自少林。北魏年间，有一药方叫少林黑膏，古称少林断续膏，是中国人长期用来治疗骨伤方面的民间验方。此药方经过少林寺武僧们千百年来的使用，对治疗风湿病、关节炎、腰腿疼痛、肩周炎、腰肌劳损、坐骨神经痛等各类骨病有康复功能。少林黑膏是传统纯手工制作的膏药，是少林寺的千年秘方，不含任何西药成分，为了保证药效，每副膏药都要经过20多道工艺，炮制时间长达2个多月，是中华传统医学宝库中的一颗明珠。目前，"少林黑膏"已被中国武术协会、中国郑州国际少林武术节作为指定用品，成为国内武术团体的馈赠礼品。

The Shaolin Temple impresses the world with its kung fu. Indeed, it has a very profound historical background and is an important part of China's traditional martial arts. Since ancient times, it has been said that the martial arts originated from Shaolin. Shaolin culture includes more than just martial arts. Shaolin orthopedics and traumatology department is also an important branch in TCM clinic. In the thousands of years of evolution, it has become such an influential school in Chinese orthopedics and traumatology that it has a parallel fame with kung fu. Shaolin black plaster, originated in the Northern Wei Dynasty, was a folk prescription used by ordinary people for a long time to treat fractures, waist and leg strain, rheumatism, and bruisism. After thousands of years of use by martial monks in the Shaolin Temple, the prescription has the rehabilitation function for various kinds of bone diseases, such as rheumatism, arthritis, pain of waist and leg, periarthritis of shoulder, strain of psoas, sciatica, etc. Shaolin black plaster is a traditional hand-made plaster, a secret recipe of the Shaolin Temple for thousands of years. To ensure its medicinal effect, each plaster has to go through more than 20 steps of processing and takes more than 2 months to complete its production, showing it is a pearl in the treasure house of traditional Chinese medicine. At present, the Chinese Martial Arts Association and Zhengzhou International Shaolin Martial Arts Festival in China have designated "Shaolin black plaster" as a gift for delegations.

# 第九节　古人洁牙妙招
## The Best Ways of Teeth Cleaning in Ancient Times

《史记·扁鹊仓公列传》记载了中国医学史上最早的齿科疾病。西汉名医淳于意用含漱苦参汤的方法治愈了齐中大夫的龋齿病。汉末三国东吴时代的高荣墓葬出土了一个小杨枝的龙形器物，研究者考证认为这是墓主人生前用来剔除齿间食物残渣的洁牙用具，也是现代牙签的雏形。隋代巢元方的《诸病源候论》也提到，饭后若不漱口便可能患上龋齿。隋唐时期的人们揩齿以保口齿清洁，有"杨枝揩齿法"和"手指揩齿法"两种。后者见于晚唐敦煌壁画中的"劳度叉斗圣图"。古人常用的漱口剂有盐水、浓茶、酒等。唐代孙思邈《千金要方》便有用盐水漱口使牙齿坚固的记载。据现代药理分析，茶叶中的单宁和氟化合物确有抗菌、预防龋齿的作用，而酒中所含的酒精有消毒作用。至于洁牙剂，或为盐或为药物散剂。而刷牙的流行则要到宋代了。两宋时期，《太平圣惠方》记载有药膏洁齿法：用柳枝、槐枝、桑枝煎水熬膏，加入姜汁、细辛等，这就是现代药物牙膏的雏形了。另据记载在宋代已经有植毛牙刷了。

The earliest dental disease in the history of Chinese medicine was recorded in the *Biography of Bian Que and Cang Gong in*

*Historical Records.* Chunyu Yi, a famous doctor in the Western Han Dynasty, cured an officer, Qi's dental caries by using the method of gargling the mouth with sophora flavescens ait liquid. A dragon-shaped twig was unearthed from the Gaorong tomb of the Eastern Wu Dynasty of the Three Kingdoms Period. Researchers believed that it was a dental cleaning tool used by the tomb owner to remove food residue between the teeth, and it is also the prototype of a modern toothpick. According to Chao Yuanfang's *Treatise on the Causes and Symptoms of Various Diseases*, dental caries may occur if one does not gargle after meals. In the Sui and Tang Dynasties, people wiped their teeth to keep them clean. There were two methods: "the poplar wiping method" and "the finger wiping method". The latter can be seen in one of Dunhuang frescoes of the late Tang Dynasty. The mouthwashes commonly used by the ancients were salt water, strong tea, liquor and so on. In the Tang Dynasty, Sun Simiao's *Valuable Prescriptions* recorded that the mouthwash with salt water was used to strengthen teeth. According to modern pharmacological analysis, tannin and fluorine compound in tea has antibacterial and preventive action of decayed teeth and alcohol in liquor has the action of disinfection. As for cleansers, they were either salt or medicinal powder. The popularization of brushing one's teeth came in the Song Dynasty. "*Taiping Shenghui Fang*" recorded the method of tooth cleaning ointment: ointment made by decocted willow branch, robinia branch and mulberry branch, then added with ginger juice, asarum, etc., which was the prototype of a modern pharmaceutical toothpaste. In addition, in the Song Dynasty there was a toothbrush with transplanted bristles.

## 第十节 桑
### Mulberry Culture

　　我国的育桑文化历史十分悠久。早在五千年前，古代先民就开始在中原大地上栽种桑树，差不多与中华民族的文明史同步。在殷商时期的甲骨文中已有"桑"字出现，秦汉以来的不少典籍中都有对桑树的描述，从战国至西汉的出土文物中也多次出现过写实的桑树形象。桑作为药用的记载，最早出现在《滇南本草》。桑的叶、果、嫩枝、根和皮都是中医临床的常用药物。桑叶能疏散风热、清肺润燥、清肝明目，可用于风热感冒、肺热燥咳、头晕头痛、目赤昏花。桑椹能滋阴补血、生津润燥，可用于肝肾阴虚、眩晕耳鸣、心悸失眠、须发早白、津伤口渴、内热消渴。桑枝能祛风湿、利关节，可用于风湿痹病，肩臂、关节酸痛麻木。桑白皮能泻肺平喘、利水消肿，可用于肺热喘咳、面目肌肤浮肿。古人食桑和栽桑养蚕差不多是同时开始的。桑文化与蚕桑文化是我国对世界物质文明和精神文明的一项重大贡献。在漫漫历史长河中，中国蚕桑文化对政治经济、社会组织、哲学宗教、文化艺术、生产生活等产生过重大的影响。

　　Our country has a long history of mulberry cultivation. As early as five thousand years ago, our ancestors began to plant mulberry trees in the Central Plain of China, almost keeping pace with the history of Chinese civilization. The Chinese character "桑" (sāng in pinyin) appeared in the inscriptions on animal bones during the Yin and Shang Dynasties. Mulberry trees has been described in many ancient books since the Qin and Han Dynasties and the realistic image of mulberry trees has appeared many times in unearthed relics from the Warring States Period to the Western Han Dynasty. Mulberry was first recorded as a medicinal herb in *Materia Medica in Southern Yunnan*. Mulberry is a big family in herbal medicine. Leaves, fruit, twigs, root and bark are commonly used in TCM clinic. Mulberry leaf can disperse wind-heat, clear away heat in the lung and liver to moisten dryness and make eyes bright, relieving dizziness and headache and congestive eyes and blurred vision. Mulberry fruit can nourish yin and blood, reinforce yin deficiency in the liver and kidney and relieve such symptoms as vertigo, tinnitus, palpitation, insomnia, early white hair, thirst. Mulberry branch can dispel wind and dampness and benefit joints. It is used for rheumatism, pain and numbness in the shoulder, arm and joint. Mulberry bark can relieve asthma due to the lung heat and benefit diuresis and eliminate facial edema. Ancient people began to eat mulberry, plant mulberry and raise silkworms at about the same time. Sericulture originated in China and made a major contribution to the material and spiritual civilization of the world. In the long history, Chinese sericulture had a great influence on politics, economy, social organization, philosophy and religion, culture and art, production and life, etc.

# 第十一节 艾
## Mugwort

灸法在中医养生治病中使用的材料并不是只有艾这一种原料，在历史上，几乎能够发热的材料人类都曾经尝试用于灸法治病中。古代资料里记载的有硫黄、黄蜡、桑枝、桃枝、灯芯草、线香等，近现代出现了电热灸、红外灸等。长时间的实践证明，艾灸具有其他灸法不能替代的独特优势，成为人们养生治病的重要手段。艾燃烧时所产生的特殊短红外线，渗透力是普通长红外线的3到4倍，对人体的渗透力在10毫米以上，能够激活细胞免疫激活素，提高人体免疫力。中医研究机构用其他药材、各种物理化学方法、射线等与艾灸做对比研究，结果没有一种方法可以完全替代艾灸。若以普通火热，则只觉皮肤表层灼痛，而没有温煦散寒的作用。艾草无处不在，田野、山冈随处可得。古人把艾草称为"百草之王"。

Mugwort is not the only material used in moxibustion. In history, almost all the materials capable of giving off heat were used in moxibustion treatment. The materials recorded in ancient times included sulfur, yellow wax, mulberry branches, peach branches, rushes and incense. In modern times, electric moxibustion and infrared moxibustion appeared. However, a long time of practice proved moxibustion with mugwort had a unique advantage that couldn't be replaced by other materials. It has become an important means for people to keep healthy and treat diseases. The special short infrared ray produced during moxibustion is 3 to 4 times as permeable as the ordinary long infrared ray. The permeable force to the human body is above 10mm, which can activate the cellular immune activator and improve the human immunity. TCM research institutions compared mugwort with other herbs, radiation, various physical and chemical methods. It turned out that there was no way to completely replace mugwort in moxibustion. Ordinary fire is so hot that it only feels burning pain without the warming and expelling cold effect. Mugwort can be found everywhere, in fields and on hills. It was hornored as "the king of grass" by the ancients.

# 第十二节　二十四节气
## The 24 Solar Terms

　　历史上中国的主要政治、经济、文化、农业活动中心多集中在黄河流域中原地区。二十四节气也就是以这一带的气候、物候为依据建立起来的。早在东周、春秋战国时期，中原劳动人民中就有了日南至、日北至的概念。人们又根据月初、月中的日月运行的位置，天气、动植物生长等自然现象，以及它们之间的关系，把一年平分为二十四等份，并且给每等份取了个专有名称，这就是二十四节气。战国后期成书的《吕氏春秋》中，就有了立春、春分、立夏、夏至、立秋、秋分、立冬、冬至等八个节气名称的记载。这八个节气，是二十四个节气中最重要的节气。标示出季节的转换，清楚地划分出一年的四季。到秦汉年间，二十四节气已完全确立。《淮南子》一书就有了和现代完全一样的二十四节气。二十四节气将天文、农事、物候和民俗实现了巧妙的结合，衍生了大量与之相关的岁时节令文化，成为中华民族传统文化的重要组成部分。至今，二十四节气对我们的生活、文化等仍有深远影响。

　　Historically, China's major political, economic, cultural and agricultural activities were mostly located in the Central Plain of the Yellow River Basin, so the 24 solar terms were established on the basis of the climate and phenology in this area. As early as the Eastern Zhou Dynasty and the Spring and Autumn and Warring States Periods, the Chinese people had the concept of Winter Solstice and Summer Solstice. According to the positions of the sun and the moon at the beginning and the middle of the month, and the natural phenomena such as the weather and the growth of plants and animals, the relationship between them, a year was then divided into twenty-four equal parts, each of which had a proper name. This is the solar term. In the late Warring States Period, there were eight solar terms such as Beginning of Spring, Spring Equinox, Start of Summer, Summer Solstice, Start of Autumn, Autumnal Equinox, Start of Winter and Winter Solstice. These eight solar terms were the most important of the twenty-four solar terms. It marked the changes of seasons and clearly identified the four seasons of the year. By the Qin and Han Dynasties, the 24 solar terms had been fully established. *Huainanzi* had the same names of the 24 solar terms as those in the modern times. The 24 solar terms combine astronomy, agriculture, phenology and folk customs in an ingenious way, giving rise to a large number of seasons related to them and making them an important part of traditional Chinese culture. The 24 solar terms are still of profound effect to our life and culture.

## （1）立春、雨水、惊蛰、春分

Start of Spring, Rain Water, Awakening of Insects, Spring Equinox

立春俗称"报春"。立春期间，气温开始上升，日照时间开始延长，降雨量开始增加。立春意味着开启一个新的轮回，是新的一年的开始。在这个节气里，人们有迎春的庆贺祭典与活动，古时候立春要祭春神，民间有吃春饼、春盘、咬萝卜等习俗。入春以后，开始吹东南风，降雨量开始增加。雨水过后，开始植树。惊蛰，气温上升，天气变暖，地下蛰伏的各种动物开始苏醒，所以古时惊蛰当日，人们会手持清香、艾草，熏家中四角，以香味驱赶蛇、虫、蚊、鼠和霉味。春分，太阳光直射赤道，地球各地的昼夜时间相等。民间有"竖蛋"的习俗。世界各地也会有数以千万计的人在做"竖蛋"试验。这一"中国习俗"，为何成了"世界游戏"，仍尚难考证。在中国岭南一带，有一个习俗，叫作"春分吃春菜"。"春菜"是一种野苋菜，长在田野中，多为嫩绿色，约有巴掌长短。采回的春菜可与鱼片"滚汤"，叫作"春汤"。

Start of Spring is commonly known as "heralding the spring". It means the increase of temperature, sunshine and rainfall and the beginning of a new cycle and a new year. In ancient times, it was a festival for the spring god. People had the custom of eating spring cakes, spring dishes, nibbling radish on this day. After the spring, the wind from southeast begins to blow and rainfall begins to increase. After Rain Water, trees are planted. Awakening of Insects symbolizes the rising temperature and warmer weather, and all sorts of animals that have been dormant underground begin to wake up. Therefore, on the day in ancient times, people would hold fragrant medicine and wormwood to smoke every room to scare away snakes, insects, mosquitoes, rats and mildew. Spring Equinox means that sunlight is directly on the equator, which equals the time of day and night in all parts of the earth. There is a folk custom of "egg balancing". Tens of millions of people around the world also experiment with "egg standing" then. How this piece of art, known as "Chinese custom", became a "world game" is still hard to know its reason. In the Lingnan area of China, there is a custom called "eating spring vegetables on Spring Equinox". "Spring vegetable" is a wild amaranth growing in the wild fields, pale green with about a palm long, which is usually made into "the soup" with fish slices.

## （2）清明、谷雨、立夏、小满、芒种、夏至

Pure Brightness, Grain Rain, Beginning of Summer, Lesser Fullness of Grain, Grain in Ear, Summer Solstice

清明时节，空气清新，草木返青，是播种的大好时光。在清明节这一天，有扫墓祭祖、踏青赏春、植树种草等传统习俗。清明既是节气又是节日。谷雨是公历每年4月20日前后，天气变暖，是播种高粱、玉米等秋作物的重要节气。立夏是夏季的开始。在我国沿海一带，立夏这一天有"斗蛋"的民俗。小满时节，农民购置农器家具，做收麦前的准备工作，并开始播种晚秋作物。在小满这一天，有"祭车神"的习俗。芒种后进入典型的夏季，天气相当炎热，麦类等有芒作物成熟。芒种这一天有"送花神"的习俗。根据古老的说法，芒种过后，群芳摇落，花神退位，人世间便要隆重地为花神饯行，以示感激。从这里，可以看出古人对大自然的一种亲近感，表现出对生态的敏感和重视。夏至是农事活动中很重要的节气，是收割小麦、秋田管理的紧张季节。

On the Qingming Day, air is fresh and the plants begin to grow. It is a good time to sow. Traditional customs such as sweeping tombs and offering sacrifices to ancestors, spring outings, planting trees and grass are practiced. Qingming is a combination of a solar term and a festival. Grain Rain is around April 20th based on the solar calendar every year. The weather is warm and is an important season for sowing sorghum, corn and other autumn crops. On Beginning of Summer, there is a folk custom of "egg fighting" in coastal areas of China. In Lesser Fullness of Grain, farmers would buy some farming furniture, do the preparatory work before the wheat is harvested, and begin to plant the late autumn crops. On this day, there is the custom of offering sacrifices to the god of the traffic tools. Grain in Ear is typical of summer with the weather quite hot. The wheat and other awn crops become mature. On this day, people have the custom of "seeing off the flower goddess". According to the old saying, the flowers will fade and the flower goddess will abdicate after Grain in Ear. People will give her a farewell dinner ceremoniously to show their gratitude. From here, we can see that the ancients had a sense of affinity to nature, showing the sensitivity and importance to ecology. Summer Solstice is a very important solar term for agriculture. It is a busy season for wheat harvesting and the management of the autumn field.

### （3）小暑、大暑、立秋、处暑、白露

Lesser Heat, Greater Heat, Beginning of Autumn, End of Heat, White Dew

小暑时节，天气逐渐炎热，汛期到来，作物生长旺盛，要加强秋作物管理。在小暑节气的前后几天，民间有"百索子撂上屋"的习俗，寄托着人们的美好愿望。大暑为一年中气温最高的时节，要注意治虫、防旱、防涝，也有"冬病夏治"的说法。在浙江台州湾一带，有"送大暑船"的习俗。清同治年间，此地常有疫病流行，尤其以大暑时节为甚。人们认为这是五位凶神所致，于是在江边建了五圣庙，还在大暑节气这一天，用特制木船将供品送至椒江口外。意思很明显，就是送走瘟疫，祈求平安。立秋，秋季开始，各种作物不能再播种了。但此时要播撒葱籽，育出小葱苗，待第二年春天移栽。还可种菠菜、青菜。立秋是农家的大节气，是庄稼接近成熟的季节。处暑，暑尽天凉，炎热的天气将在这日结束。在处暑时节，正值农历七月十五前后，民间会有庆赞中元的民俗活动，俗称"做七月半"或"中元节"。台湾也有"拜好兄弟"的习俗。白露，时值中秋，天气转凉，夜间露水发白，开始收获高粱和早玉米。

Lesser Heat means weather gradually gets hot and floods are frequent. Crops start to grow and people will do the farm work.

Greater Heat is the hottest time of the year. Attention should be paid to insect control, drought control and water logging control. There is a saying that "winter ailments are treated in summer". In Taizhou Bay, Zhejiang Province, there is the custom of "bidding ships of Great Heat farewell". During the reign of Emperor Tongzhi in the Qing Dynasty, epidemics were frequent, especially in the season of Greater Heat. People believed they were caused by the five evil gods, so they built five holy temples by the river. On the day of Greater Heat, special wooden boats were used to send the offerings to the outside of the mouth of the Jiaojiang River. The obvious meaning was to send away the plague and pray for peace. Start of Autumn means autumn begins and all kinds of crops can't be planted any more. But at this time, people sow scallion seeds and cultivate young scallion seedlings in order to be transplanted next spring. Start of Autumn is a big solar term for local farmers. It is the season when crops are nearly ripe. End of Heat means the hot weather will end on this day. During the End of Heat season, when it is around the 15th day of the 7th lunar month, there will be folk activities to celebrate Zhongyuan Festival. In Taiwan Province, there is the custom of "worshiping good brothers". White Dew, which is around the Mid-autumn day, means the weather turns cool and the dew turns whitish at night. People begin to harvest sorghum and early corn.

## （4）秋分、寒露、霜降、立冬、小雪、大雪

Autumn Equinox, Cold Dew, Frost's Descent, Start of Winter,
Lesser Snow, Greater Snow

秋分是传统的"祭月节"。我国自古就有"春祭日、秋祭月"的说法。我们现在庆祝的中秋节则是由传统的"祭月节"发展而来。据考证，最初"祭月节"是定在"秋分"这一天，不过由于这一天在农历八月里的日子每年不同，不一定都有圆月，而祭月无圆月则会大煞风景。所以，人们就将"祭月节"由"秋分"调至中秋。进入寒露，气候明显转凉，夜有寒冷之感。寒露节气宜人的气候十分适合登山，慢慢地重阳节登高的习俗也成了寒露时节的习俗。霜降，以天冷、露水结成薄霜而名。立冬，意味着冬天的到来，是作物收割后要收藏起来的意思。小雪时节，气温下降，此时开始农田水利基本建设，整修道路，开展副业活动。每年的这个时候，大人和孩子们都会在嘴上唠叨着：几号了，还有几天就要到小雪了，谁家的糯米碾好了，谁家的还在场上晒着呢。这时候小孩子们都很兴奋，觉得就像过年似的。大雪，因天寒地冻、大雪纷飞而名。农事活动继续以水利建设、整修道路水渠为主，并开始磨粉，制作粉条、粉皮，从事商业经营及商品生产等活动。

Autumn Equinox is the traditional festival of offering sacrifices to the moon. Since ancient times, China has had "offering sacrifices to the sun in the spring and the moon in the autumn". The modern Mid-autumn Festival came from the traditional festival of offering sacrifices to the moon. It is believed that the festival was originally held on the Autumn Equinox day when there was not always a full moon because the date of the festival varied from year to year in the eighth lunar month. If weather is bad, fun will be spoiled if there is no moon to be worshiped on that day absolutely. Later on, the "festival of worshiping the moon" shifted from "Autumn Equinox" to the Mid-autumn Festival. Entering Cold Dew, the climate obviously turned cool. People will feel cold at night. The pleasant climate of Cold Dew is very suitable for mountaineering, and the custom of climbing mountains on the Double Ninth Festival has become the custom of the Cold Dew seasons. Frost's Descent is known as a thin frost formed by cold weather and dew. Start of Winter, the coming of winter, means collecting crops after they are harvested. Lesser Snow means temperature drops. People begin with irrigation and water conservancy construction, road repair and sideline activities. At this time of a year, both adults and children will talk about the crop harvest of a year. Children are very excited, because another New Year is coming around. Greater Snow means heavy snow. Agricultural activities continue to focus on water conservancy construction, repairing roads and canals and begin to mill powder, the production of vermicelli. People engage in activities such as business and commodity production.

## （5）冬至、小寒、大寒

## Winter Solstice, Lesser Cold, Greater Cold

冬至兼具自然与人文两大内涵，既是自然节气，也是一个传统的祭祀祖先和神灵的节日。古人认为自冬至起，天地阳气渐强，代表下一个循环开始，是大吉之日。在中国的北方地区，每年农历冬至这天，不论家境贫富，饺子是必不可少的。这个习俗的由来，是因为纪念"医圣"张仲景冬至舍药留下的。小寒，进入严寒天气，梅花是小寒节气的第一花信，梅花自古就是诗人们咏赞不衰的题材。咏梅诗起源于六朝，隋唐时崛起，极盛于宋元，明清相继，仍余韵犹存。这些诗词或写梅品质，或咏梅风姿，或绘梅神韵，或歌梅情怀，大都立意新颖，借傲霜斗雪、不畏严寒的梅花以抒发作者不畏强暴、敢于斗争的高尚情操。大寒，进入一年中最寒冷的时段，时在农历十二月，准备过春节。在大寒节气中，其间有一个对于北方人非常重要的日子——腊八，即阴历腊月初八。在这一天，人们用五谷杂粮加上花生、栗子、红枣、莲子等熬成一锅香甜美味的"腊八粥"。腊八粥有和胃、补脾、养心、清肺、益肾、利肝、明目、安神、通便等作用，即可增强人体免疫力，又可耐寒。

Winter Solstice has both natural and cultural connotations. It is not only a natural solar term, but also a traditional festival for offering sacrifices to ancestors and gods. The ancient believed that since Winter Solstice, yang in nature has become stronger, which represented the beginning of the next cycle and marked the auspicious day. In northern China, jiaozi (dumplings) is an essential holiday food for both rich and poor families on the annual Winter Solstice. The origin of this custom is to commemorate the "medical saint" Zhang Zhongjing who dispensed medicine to the sick on Winter Solstice. Lesser Cold is a sign of entering the cold weather, in which plum blossom is the first sign. Plum blossom has been a popular theme for poets since ancient times. It originated in the Six Dynasties, rose in the Sui and Tang dynasties, flourished in the Song and Yuan Dynasties, and survived in the Ming and Qing dynasties. These poems were about the implication and graceful charm of plum, expressing poets' admiration and the noble sentiment of bravery like the quality of plum. Greater Cold, the coldest time of the year, is in the 12th lunar month. People begin to prepare for the Spring Festival. Laba, or the eighth day of the twelfth lunar month, is a very important day for people in the north during Greater Cold. On this day, people will make a pot of sweet and delicious "Laba porridge" with various grains plus peanuts, chestnuts, red dates, lotus seeds and so on. It can tonify and nourish the five-zang organs and benefit vision and defecation with an improved ability of immunity and anti-cold.

# 第十三节　香　俗
## Incense Custom

　　焚香是旧时民俗。敬天地、祖宗要焚香，面对神佛、仙家要焚香，祛邪避秽要焚香，还有焚香拜月抚琴、焚香读书，几乎无处不焚香。室内焚香，也叫熏香，多是为了清洁房间和衣被，除湿、杀虫、避秽。室内熏香的习俗，早在战国时代已经出现。但当时所焚之香，多为草本植物，熏香时，将香草置于香炉中直接点燃，香味不浓，且烟较大。西汉时，中外交通和贸易往来更加频繁，东南亚和西亚一带的香料开始输入。熏香的习俗由此更加广为流行。唐代是中国焚香习俗的鼎盛时期。从文献记载看，唐朝时期的各个阶层的人的生活都离不开焚香，熏香已经成为人们生活的一部分。宋代大量进口香料，除部分入药和用于礼佛外，主要供给宫廷、官宦之家日常使用。一些香料经过几百年的历史过程，从传入之初作为焚香原料，用来供拜神佛之类信仰民俗活动，逐渐而演变成治病的方药。经过了漫长的文化整合，被吸收到中华本草大家庭，并且产生了大量疗效确切的方剂和中成药。

　　Burning incense was an important event in the folk life in old days. Chinese burned incense to worship their ancestors, heaven and earth, the moon and the gods, to remove evil spirits, even when they played a musical instrument, read books and so on. Indoor incense was mostly used to keep rooms and clothes away from peculiar odor, wetness, insects, etc. The custom of indoor incense first appeared in the Warring States Period. But at that time herbs were used as burned materials which had dense smoke and little fragrance. During the Western Han Dynasty, trade between China and foreign countries became more frequent and spices from Southeast Asia and West Asia began to be imported. The custom of burning incense became even more popular. The Tang Dynasty was the heyday of incense burning in China. From the literature records, burning incense had been a necessary part in people's life in the Tang Dynasty. In the Song Dynasty, a large number of spices were imported, which were mainly used for the daily life of the court and officials, except for some medicinal use and Buddha ritual. Hundreds of years later, some spices, from the beginning of the introduction of incense as raw materials for worshipping Buddha evolved into medicine to cure diseases. After a long period of cultural integration, it was absorbed into the big family of Chinese Materia Medica and a large number of effective prescriptions and proprietary Chinese medicines were created.

## 第十四节　重阳登高
## Mountain Climbing on the Double Ninth Festival

关于重阳节登高的由来流传着一个有趣的说法。据说东汉时汝南一带瘟魔为害，疫病流行。有一个叫桓景的人，拜道长费长房为师，学消灾救人的法术。一天，费长房告诉桓景，九月初九，瘟魔又要来害人，并嘱咐桓景回去搭救乡亲："九日离家登高，把茱萸装入红布袋，扎在胳膊上，喝菊花酒，就能战胜瘟魔"。桓景回家，遍告乡亲。九月初九，汝河汹涌澎湃，瘟魔来犯，但因菊花酒刺鼻，茱萸香刺心，难以接近百姓。桓景便挥剑斩瘟魔于山下。傍晚，人们返回家园，见家中鸡犬牛羊，都暴死，而人们因出门登高而免受灾殃。自此，重阳登高避灾流传至今。久而久之，登高便变成了一个美好、风雅的习俗。另一传说说的是重阳时节，秋收已经完毕，农事相对比较空闲。这时山野里的野果、药材之类正是成熟的季节，农民纷纷上山采集，从此演变成登高的风俗。此外，重阳节期间天气晴朗，气温凉爽，也适合人们登高望远。

There is an interesting legend about the origin of climbing mountains on the Double Ninth Festival. It is said that the epidemic raged in Runan area in ancient times. There was a man named Huan Jing, the student of Fei Zhangfang, a Taoist who had the magic of eliminating disasters and saving people. One day, Fei Zhangfang told Huan Jing that on the ninth day of the ninth lunar month, the pestilent devil would attack someone again. He told Huan Jing to go back and rescue his fellow villagers, telling them that they should leave home to climb up the hill, put the dogwood in a red cloth bag, tie it on their arms and drink chrysanthemum liquor on that day. Huan Jing went home and told all his fellow villagers about it. On the 9th day of the 9th lunar month, the river surged with the evil spirit of pestilence existing, but it was hard to get close because of the pungent chrysanthemum liquor and the fierce fragrance of the dogwood. Huan Jing killed the devil in the mountain with his sword. In the evening, people returned to their homes and found their livestock-chickens, dogs, cattle and sheep were all killed, but villagers were saved. Since then, the Double Ninth Hill-climbing custom has spread to today. As time went on, climbing a mountain became a beautiful and elegant custom. Another story about the Double Ninth Festival is when the autumn harvest was over, people were relieved from farming affairs. At this time the wild fruits, medicinal materials and the like in the mountains were ripe, farmers went up a mountain to collect them. The custom of climbing mountains probably evolved from that. Besides, it was sunny and cool during the Double Ninth Festival, which was suitable for climbing high and looking far away.

## 第十五节 椒房殿
### Pepper Hall

椒房殿是中国古代传统的宫殿建筑，在西汉都城长安城内，属未央宫建筑群，是皇后居住的地方。之所以命名为椒房殿是因为宫殿的墙壁上使用花椒树的花朵及其果皮所制成的粉末进行粉刷。花椒药性辛温，有散寒、温中、杀虫、祛湿的作用，用它刷墙，有祛邪防病保暖保健的功效。刷了花椒粉的墙呈粉色，有一股芳香的味道，而且这样做还可以保护木质结构，可以防蛀虫。又一说，因为花椒树多籽，人们取它"多子"的含义，希望皇后子嗣繁盛，多半是皇室成员们的美好愿望。相传窦漪房窦皇后在世时，常常在椒房殿里休息，墙壁上的花椒粉末对人有好处，因此窦皇后在世时间也很长，身体健康不说，还为自己的丈夫汉文帝，为自己的儿子汉景帝做了不少事。汉高祖七年（公元前200年）长乐宫建成，刘邦从临时都城栎阳搬到长安入住长乐宫，这时吕雉为皇后住在长乐宫的椒房殿；汉惠帝（公元前195年－公元前188年在位）即位后未央宫基本建成，从此皇后如张嫣、窦漪房、陈阿娇、卫子夫等都居住过未央宫的椒房殿。

Pepper Hall is an ancient Chinese traditional palace building, which belongs to the Weiyang Palace complex and is the residence of the empresses in Chang'an, the capital of the Western Han Dynasty.

The reason why it is named Pepper Hall is that the walls of the palace are painted with the powder made from the flowers and fruit peels of wild pepper trees. The warm and pungent property of the powder has the effect of dispersing cold, warming the middle energizer, repelling pests, dispelling the pathogenic factors and preventing diseases. The wall color is pink with a fragrant odor, which can protect the wooden structure from moth damage. Another view is that Chinese pepper ash has many seeds, which is associated with an auspicious implication of "many children" in Chinese culture. Pepper Hall seems to be equipped with the heating system due to its property. Legend has it that when the Empress Dou Yifang was alive, she often took a rest in the Hall of Pepper. The prickly ash powder on the wall was so beneficial to her health that she lived a long life and supported her husband, Emperor Wen and her son, Emperor Jing of the Han Dynasty a lot. In the seventh year of Emperor Gaozu of the Han Dynasty (200 B.C.), Changle Palace was built, when Liu Bang moved from the temporary capital Yueyang to Chang'an and settled in it. At that time, Lu Zhi, the empress, lived in Pepper Hall. After Emperor Hui of the Han Dynasty (195 B.C. — 188 B.C.) came to the throne, the Weiyang Palace was basically completed. From then on, queens such as Zhang Yan, Dou Yifang, Chen Ajiao and Wei Zifu ever lived in Pepper Hall of Weiyang Palace.

## 第十六节 素 食
### A Vegetarian Diet

如果看一部吃的历史，素食是其中一直涌动的潜流。最早的人是吃素食的。钻木取火这一方法普及之前，吃肉对人的身体伤害极大。因此，在学会食品再加工之前，只吃素食。在有肉吃的情况下，能够意识到素食的重要，最早见于《吕氏春秋》。汉朝人有很多素食可吃，因为在汉代，引进了一大堆蔬菜瓜果，大大增加了素食的食材品种。最伟大的素食也是在汉朝发明的。这个功劳与淮南王刘安有关。刘安爱炼丹，并且有一定的名声，也恰恰因为这个爱好，无意间炼出了最伟大的素食——豆腐。据考证豆腐在汉朝其实远没有普及，技术也不成熟，其凝固性和口感与唐宋的豆腐没法比，因此还进不了烹饪主流。直到唐宋，豆腐才成了重要的素食。唐朝时还随鉴真东渡传到日本，日本人也学会了做豆腐。北宋首都汴梁已经有了专做素食的菜馆，南宋首都临安流行的素食有上百种。素食登峰造极是在清代，形成了流派和理论。

Vegetarianism has always been around ever since man existed on this planet. Before the popularization of fire, eating raw meat was very harmful to human body. They ate only vegetarian food because they didn't know how to process raw meat. Later, with the cooked meat popular in human, ancient Chinese people didn't neglect the importance of vegetarian foods, which was cited from the record of more than 2,000 years ago. There were a lot of vegetarian foods in the Han Dynasty because a large number of fruits and vegetables were introduced from other countries. It is recorded that the greatest vegetarian diet was also invented in the Han Dynasty. This credit has something to do with Liu An, the king of Huainan in the Han Dynasty. Liu An loved alchemy and had a certain reputation for it. It is precisely because of this hobby, he inadvertently produced the greatest vegetarian food: tofu. According to research, tofu was far from popular in the Han Dynasty because its processing technology was not mature then. Its solidification and taste could not be compared with those in the Tang and Song dynasties, so it could not enter the mainstream of cooking then. It was not until the Tang and Song dynasties that tofu became an important vegetarian food. During the Tang Dynasty, Jianzhen traveled east to Japan, where the Japanese learned to make tofu. There were vegetarian restaurants in Bianliang, the capital of the Northern Song Dynasty. Vegetarian dishes with a wide variety became popular in Lin'an, the capital of the Southern Song Dynasty. Vegetarianism reached its peak in the Qing Dynasty, forming various schools and theories.

## 第十七节 孔子的饮食养生
### Confucius's Dietary Regimen

　　孔子一生大部分时间不得志，经历了许多生活纷扰，可是他仍活了72岁。应该说，孔子是长寿的，这与他晚年注重饮食有关。孔子的"八不食"理论为医家所推崇，具体是：腐烂变质的食物，颜色和气味不正的食物，烹调方法不当的食物，不合时令的食物，以及超过三天的祭祀用肉都不能食用。孔子关于饮食的论述可谓全面系统，其标准之高即便是我们在今天看来也未必能够完全达到。其实，在对饮食的高标准之下，更多的是对自身欲望和行为的节制。不放纵口腹之欲，有节制地享受美食，是孔子饮食养生的要旨，值得现代人借鉴。以姜酒佐餐，但勿多食。从中医的角度，酒可活血通络，姜可暖胃驱寒，但过量则会伤身。孔子的见解还有崇尚节俭、遵从礼节的考虑。

　　Confucius was unsuccessful for most of his life and experienced a lot of ups and downs, but he had a 72-year lifespan which was a long life at his time. Probably it has something to do with his dietary habit in his later years. In Confucius's diet, eight foods are inedible. These include: food that has gone bad and changed its original color or smell; food that is not cooked properly; unseasonable food; sacrificial meat over three days. Confucius's dietary habit was strict and systematic that even today we may not be able to reach it completely. In fact, it is more about the moderation of one's own desires and behaviors. It is the essence of Confucius' diet to keep healthy: no indulgence in appetite and moderation in food. Take ginger and liquor as example, they are good accompaniment to a meal but don't take them too much. From the point of view of TCM, liquor can activate blood circulation and ginger can warm the stomach and keep cold away, but overeating them will hurt the body. To some extent, Confucius practised frugality and etiquette.